Reaching for Normal

Reaching for Normal

*A Mother's Memoir of Raising
a Child with Brain Cancer
and Chronic Illness*

AMY DANIELS

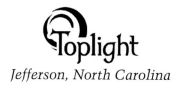

Jefferson, North Carolina

ISBN (print) 978-1-4766-8535-9
ISBN (ebook) 978-1-4766-4284-0

LIBRARY OF CONGRESS AND BRITISH LIBRARY
CATALOGUING DATA ARE AVAILABLE

Front cover image Emily and I just received
our gift of a trip to Disney World,
photograph by Jeff Daniels.
Background © 2021 Shutterstock

Printed in the United States of America

Toplight is an imprint of McFarland & Company, Inc., Publishers

*Box 611, Jefferson, North Carolina 28640
www.toplightbooks.com*

To my world
Dave, Emily, and *Ryan*

Acknowledgments

Emily has guided me through my life for the past two decades. She's the one who made me a mom and challenged me beyond any expectation. She has also taught me the most, including how to keep on smiling. Ryan, words can't express the joy and the comfort you bring to our family. Thank you for your reminders of normalcy, laughter, and patience, especially as I wrote this book. Mom and Dad, your endless love and support for me and my family has never gone unnoticed. Thank you. Kim, my skinny bitch, thank you for cheering me on and for always being available to help take care of Em. Mike, thank you for never wavering in being there for me and my family and for being the kids' favorite uncle. Jeff, no matter where you are in the world, you show up. Thank you for also being the kids' favorite uncle and for providing our family with Sara and the boys. Katie and Christopher, the best examples of cousin love, thank you for sharing your parents with us throughout the years. Tammy, thank you for always being there. And to Dave, my biggest supporter, provider of laughter, and believer in me—thank you for your encouragement to write these words and letting me share our story.

I would also like to thank the early readers of my memoir, especially Steph and Uncle Paul, for your valuable input. And finally, thank you Toplight Books for working with me to publish it.

Table of Contents

Table of Contents

Preface

Being a parent to a child who has a chronic illness and disability can feel overwhelmingly lonely. I hope this book brings a familiar, relatable story to other parents who face similar challenges and therefore makes them feel less alone in their journey. More, though, I hope others can find interest in, and maybe even relate to, this story—bridging the gap between "typical" families and "special" families. I would love for the reader to understand that we are not all that different, although our experiences may be different—most of us find the same joys and challenges in life.

This is a true story. I have changed the names of some of the people in the book for privacy reasons.

≋ 1 ≋

The Diagnosis

"Your daughter has a brain tumor." Those were the six words that changed my life.

Up until I heard those words, I was your typical overzealous first-time mom juggling a career and motherhood. I was living in my cute, yet run-down, starter home with my husband of four years in the middle of suburbia. As soon as I found out I was pregnant I started eating obnoxiously healthy foods, swore off all coffee and alcohol, walked daily for exercise and read all about pregnancy and babies instead of going out on the weekends. And once our daughter was born, my husband and I continued to be obnoxiously healthy and did things like read novels aloud to the baby and listen to classical music to better her development. Dave, on par with our peers, changed most of the diapers, helped with the midnight feedings and juggled that with his job.

But then those words.

Emily was seven months old. We had been going to the doctor's office more than usual over the course of the last several months because it became apparent that she didn't act quite the same as the other babies we read about in the books. It was a slow process as she was our first baby and we were, admittedly, clueless. Yes, she cried, and cried, and cried, and she never slept. But babies did that, right? Those were the horror stories we had heard. *Get ready for no sleep! Be prepared to leave the restaurant because the baby is crying!*

Emily was our porcelain doll baby—fair skin, light blue eyes disproportionately big for her petite face, and a head with just a touch of blonde peach fuzz. She was my beautiful everything. We were just like our friends with new babies; she was all we could talk about. *How*

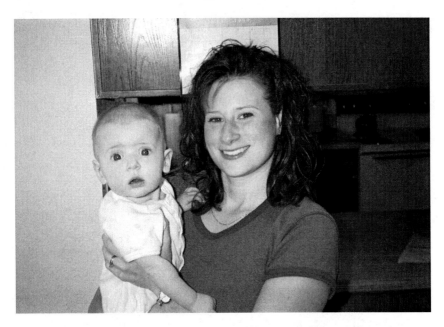

Me just before my 26th birthday and Emily, age five months (before her diagnosis).

did your baby sleep last night? Oh, your baby graduated to size two diapers? Our everyday lives—work, owning our first home, pets—all became secondary. Our life then, both for us and for all our friends, revolved around our infants.

"Emily," we laughed to the outside world, "is just a high maintenance baby." Dave and I knew about the feeding schedule. We knew how much babies were supposed to sleep. We knew every milestone and when it should be reached. After all, it seemed we read every book published on what to do with a new baby. We tried to laugh about our child shrieking and demanding bottles that she didn't drink. "Such a strong-willed, independent little lady!" But we also avoided taking her out to the grocery store or post office or restaurants. You just never knew when she would start screaming.

My mother-in-law came to visit when Emily was just weeks old. She was a whiz with kids, from babies to teens. She raised four of her own and worked with special needs children in the local elementary school. And I couldn't wait for her visit to show off my bundle of joy. Predictably, throughout each day of my mother-in-law's stay, Emily screamed her typical 20-minute ear-piercing crying sessions. With each fit, we just shrugged and did our passing her around, burping, feeding, rocking routine. By now this was a multiple-times-a-day act for us. But my mother-in-law, shaking her head, said, "She's crying like she's in pain. Babies don't usually sound like that. Maybe the formula isn't agreeing with her." With that, we made an appointment with the doctor. I was hopeful that my mother-in-law was right about the formula. I was ready for the screaming to stop.

The first pediatrician we saw conducted his physical exam and agreed as she shrieked when he looked in her eyes and ears. "She's acting like something is bothering her," he said. "I can't find anything wrong, though." Emily, now settled, sat propped in my arms and gazed at the doctor with her piercing blue eyes and played with his tie. There was nothing out of the ordinary going on by the end of his exam.

But the crying and not eating continued. So we went back to the doctor's office several weeks later when Emily was three months old and saw a new pediatrician. The second pediatrician said, "She's probably allergic to milk." Just like my mother-in-law thought! We immediately thought highly of this young pediatrician after his quick diagnosis. With that, he advised us to start using a specialized formula that contained no dairy products. Although happy for a possible end to the sleepless nights and cry fests, we slowly went broke paying for this formula. I often wondered if it was laced with gold given the price, but, like any parents, we would pay whatever it was to make Emily happy (and for us to get some sleep).

We tried the new formula and didn't notice any difference in Emily's mood. The crying continued and she still would only have an ounce or two of formula at a time. I was still operating on the amount of sleep a parent with a newborn has, even though Emily was now five months old and (according to the books) should have been sleeping through the night. I was certain my blood flowed dark brown, the color of coffee.

My husband and I shared child-rearing duties equally. Dave went to work three days a week (12½-hour shifts), and I worked part-time at the university on the days he was home. We both had stay-at-home moms growing up and it was important to us to provide that home environment for Emily. However, being able to afford to eat was also important to us, so we were lucky that we each had jobs that allowed one of us to be home every day. On multiple occasions, though, I would receive phone calls at work from Dave that made my heart sink.

"She's screaming again and won't stop. I can't do anything to make her stop. God, I hate this."

My mood quickly deteriorated. I wanted to swoop in and try to make Emily stop crying.

"She's probably tired. I was up with her again most of the night," I calmly suggested, trying to diffuse his mood and give Emily a pass.

"Well, she's in her crib. I had to put her in there and walk away. She's still screaming. She can sleep or not, but I can't stand the crying anymore. I'm done."

"I'll try to get out of here and come home," I responded, unable to bear the fact that he was so frustrated, and I was helpless sitting at my desk.

He protested, "Don't! You don't need to come home. She'll cry whether you're here or not."

My heart still in my stomach, though, I thought of an excuse to leave work early so I could rescue both Emily and Dave. When I walked through the door at home, Dave rolled his eyes and shook his head. And Emily was asleep in her crib. The stress in our relationship was mounting.

In between the moments of tension, when Emily would scream and we couldn't console her, she was content—smiling and even laughing as we gazed at her. Many times, in fact. Dave read countless books to her and she would sit in his lap, enraptured by both the pictures and the sound of his voice. I spent hours pacing the floors of our house with Emily, swaying to Tracy Chapman songs on repeat, savoring the smell of her baby-shampooed head as she leaned on my shoulder.

When Emily was six months old, we took her on a four-hour flight from our home in Colorado to Connecticut to visit both sets of our parents. She was no crankier than most other babies, it seemed, both on the flight and on our vacation. "She's out of her routine," we said to explain the screaming fits and wasted bottles to others. Dave's sister, Tammy, swayed and rocked her hours at a time— we called it the "Tammy Rock"—and inevitably she would get our high-maintenance baby to fall asleep several nights on that trip.

Once home, I would try to mimic her magical moves to get Emily to stop screaming.

After the trip, Emily was still drinking the pricey formula and still having sleepless nights. I was failing at the Tammy Rock. We then noticed that when there was a toy next to her right hand, she would reach over with her left hand to grab it—her right hand not moving. When she was in her bouncy chair, she would make it rock by kicking her left leg. Always just her left leg. After I explained this to my mom, she said, "I think you should take her to a physical therapist to see if there are exercises to do to get her to use her right side."

Back to the doctor we went for a referral to physical therapy. At this point, I wanted to stress to him that I wasn't one of *those* first-time moms. It wasn't my intention to bring Emily in for every little thing. But here we were in the little white room with cheerful flowers and posters on healthy eating on the wall with the pediatrician examining her, looking for something that was making Emily not eat, not use her right hand, and cry a high-pitched cry. Again.

The doctor explained, in an impatient and condescending tone, "She's just a stubborn lefty with a small belly. You need to force her to use her right hand by restraining her left and be really consistent with her feeding schedule."

In other words, I internalized, it was my fault she was like this. Maybe I *was* one of those first-time moms who brought their kid to the doctor for every little thing. I was a young twenty-six-year-old, deer-in-the-headlights, first-time mom who not only knew nothing about babies but was screwing this one up.

Although now thoroughly embarrassed and ashamed about bringing her in for this appointment, I went ahead and asked for a referral to physical therapy. Really, what else did I have to lose? Besides, I knew my mom would be adamant that we take her to see one. With a patronizing smirk, the pediatrician literally threw the piece of paper with the referral into my lap, saying, while shaking his head, "She really doesn't need physical therapy." With tears of both anger and shame, I left the office with a crying baby but referral in hand.

We had to wait a few weeks before our appointment with the physical therapist, so we tried the doctor's suggestion to restrain Emily's left arm, forcing her to use her right arm. We got her dressed in a onesie but didn't pull her left arm through the arm hole, keeping it stuck under the shirt. Emily instantly got upset and we waited for her right arm to move. After watching her struggle for several minutes without seeing any movement, I pulled her arm free.

"The doctor told us to do this," Dave sighed, clearly frustrated that I just gave up.

"It's barbaric. I can't stand to see her struggle like that. Look how upset it's making her," I pleaded.

"You're being too soft with her. She needs to learn to use her right hand," he gently tried explaining to me. Dave tried again with her when I wasn't around, and when I found out it made me so upset that I couldn't look at him.

"How could you do that to her?" I screamed at him.

"I'm just doing what the doctor told us to do!" Dave shouted back.

We spent much of Emily's first months arguing about the best way to take care of her. Dave would accuse me of feeding her a bottle any time she fussed, blaming me for the fact she wouldn't drink a full bottle at a sitting. I would be angry at Dave when he let her catnap too much during the day, thinking that was why she was up for hours in the middle of the night. She was miserable so often; it became easy to blame each other for creating this monster that cried all the time.

We threatened divorce multiple times before Emily was six months old. How quickly we lost that feeling of love and infatuation we felt during our college days. I fell hard and fast for Dave during my first few weeks on campus. He was intelligent, funny, and outgoing—always the life of the party. The opposite of me. I was reserved and quiet. So timid, in fact, I couldn't muster up the courage to live at college after I graduated from high school, opting instead to go to the university located a few minutes from my house, living in the safety of home with my parents. Dave, in stark contrast, drove himself to that university on his freshman move-in day a few years earlier and confidently settled into dorm life all on his own.

A mutual friend had introduced me to Dave during my first week of school. I continued to run into him multiple times on campus and each time he easily chatted with me. Within weeks, I got up the nerve to attend a party he and his roommates were hosting, after much convincing from Dave, and couldn't wait to go back for more.

The fun he was having was infectious. Although I was self-conscious of my shyness, he told me he appreciated my quiet ways, always seemingly deep in thought. We were a bit of a disparity—he loud and brash, me quiet and polite. But we shared the same core values which bonded us quickly. We spent many nights in our early years talking into the wee hours of the morning discussing current events, cultural norms, and, eventually, our dreams for our future together. I started to let my guard down. I became a bit more outgoing, although no one would accuse me of being gregarious.

During one of our late-night talks, I told Dave about a trip out west I took with my parents when I was in high school. I was taken with the landscape—so different than my surroundings in the Northeast. I shared with Dave my desire to explore more and to go back west. Dave said that he, too, would love to travel and see the world. And that sealed it. Right after we graduated from college, we got married. A few months later, we started our exploration adventure by quitting the jobs that got us through college and moved to Colorado, where my older brother and his family had recently moved. With Dave by my side, I was finally confident enough to leave my parents.

We somehow managed to survive being jobless and friendless in a new area—perhaps the naivety and optimism of being young was on our side. We lived in an old apartment with furniture we found in the building's dumpster, proudly using it with no shame. In between searching for jobs, we spent our time hiking the beautiful Rocky Mountains. Not only was it a great way to explore the area, get fresh air, and exercise, it was one of the only activities we could afford. Fortunately, we found jobs that sparked our careers within months of moving to Colorado. Three years later, during which we were entirely loving our Colorado life—working, hiking, skiing and traveling throughout the west—we had saved enough money for a down payment on a house in the Denver suburbs. We furnished it with furniture this time bought at a department store. A little while later, we learned I was pregnant with a healthy baby girl.

I didn't think we were all that different experiencing the cracks in our marital foundation as we wandered through this new world of parenting for the first time. Our friends confided in us that they, too, were treading on new ground trying to balance the needs of their babies with their relationships. After most blow-ups that resulted in a threat of divorce, Dave and I would eventually admit that we were just extremely tired and that, of course, the other was a good parent. And if we couldn't muster those words, we avoided each other by going to work on our respective days and talked minimally, barely giving each other a glance. We just went through the motions of the days—working and taking care of Emily.

Finally, the time came to take Emily to her physical therapy appointment. The waiting room was filled with other parents and kids who were wearing braces or in wheelchairs. I suddenly felt awkward and out of place wasting an appointment time with my child whose only diagnosis was stubbornness. But the hope that the physical therapist would have the answer needed to make Emily use her right hand pushed me to walk through the room and find a chair to wait in. I put Emily on my lap. Twenty long minutes later, relief set in as a perky young physical therapist with a big smile warmly welcomed us back to the gym.

After I explained that Emily didn't use her right hand or leg, the therapist examined Emily for about five minutes and asked, "What is her neurological diagnosis?"

I laughed and said, "Oh no, she's fine—just doesn't use her right side."

She then asked, "Has she had any neurological testing done?"

I said no and reiterated what the pediatrician told me ... again saying she is fine.

With a look of confusion, she said, "But I can't feel any reflexes on her right side."

I stared back at her blankly.

"She probably has some sort of neurological condition going on causing her to only use one side of her body. She needs a test done, like an MRI, to find out," the therapist gently explained. I sensed a bit of urgency from the therapist. It seemed serious, but I didn't know, and I didn't know what to ask.

With my permission, she called the pediatrician and relayed her findings along with a need for Emily to have further testing, and our session ended.

I called my mom after that visit to ask what the therapist meant by "neurological condition." I blamed the fact that I hadn't slept through the night in seven months for my not being able to understand seemingly simple terminology. My mom didn't hide the concern in her voice when she explained, "It means there is something wrong with her neurological system—her brain or spine. You need to get her to a pediatric neurologist immediately."

I got off the phone and started pacing. When Dave got home from work, I told him about the visit with the physical therapist and he rapidly fired questions at me. *What do you mean 'wrong with her brain'? Or spine? Can it be fixed? Is she in pain?* I stopped thinking; my head went into the sand like an ostrich. "I don't know" was all I could mutter, over and over again.

Within the week, we had a referral to the Children's Hospital neurology clinic. This time it was easy to get a referral from the pediatrician since the physical therapist had called him with her findings. And although I felt vindicated, thinking back to how the pediatrician made me feel initially, I was nervous and confused. This would be the first of many times I had a feeling of winning for losing. I didn't understand what lay ahead. The hope of finding out and fixing what might be causing Emily to not use her right hand, though, made me move forward with optimistic urgency. Dave and I immediately grew more patient with Emily (and each other), now beginning to understand that perhaps it wasn't our fault she was so unhappy.

Emily cried so hard she passed out when the neurologist examined her. Taking advantage of the silence, the neurologist explained, "Yes, she most likely has a neurological problem. Her history, along with my exam of her, especially when I looked in her eyes, makes me certain of this." He went on to explain, "Cerebral palsy, a stroke, or a brain tumor cause the types of symptoms she's been exhibiting. In this case, though, I'm 99.5% certain that she has cerebral palsy—like a small scar on her brain that is causing her not to use her right side."

"What?" I asked him, not truly believing what I just heard. I don't know what I was expecting to hear, maybe I was just hopeful that he would say she was perfectly fine. She's just indeed stubborn.

Tears sprang to my eyes as he repeated the words "cerebral palsy," "stroke," and "brain tumor." I couldn't look at Dave, the shock of this news paralyzing me with my eyes locked on Emily, still passed out on the exam table. I finally looked at the doctor who smiled widely and reassured us, "With proper physical and occupational therapy, she'll regain the use of her limbs and you'd never even know she had this diagnosis by the time she's in kindergarten." He went on in a calming voice, "Her case is so minor and she's young. She'll retrain her brain and the most she'll have is a slight limp. Most people won't even know." With this I relaxed, and my eyes stopped tearing. She could get better. *What naïve relief I felt at hearing that news.*

The neurologist ordered an MRI to be done the next week so he could see the size of the so-called scar on her brain. "The MRI is just a tool I'm going to use to help me better understand the severity, or lack thereof, of the damage." He went on to say, "This is a test that you don't need to be concerned about—the results would likely mean nothing to you. But I'll call you a few days after the MRI with my findings."

The appointment ended and we walked, without speaking, down the long corridor to the parking garage with Dave carrying Emily in her car seat carrier. "I don't know what to think," Dave said, finally breaking the silence.

"I was terrified at first, but I'm okay now. Once he said that no one would even know she has cerebral palsy by the time she's five, I felt better," I said, already feeling the pressure of wanting my child to fit in.

"But he said he wasn't even positive it was cerebral palsy. What else did he say it could be?"

"A stroke or a brain tumor. He was 99.5% certain it was cerebral palsy, though," I snapped. I could tell by Dave's tone that he was questioning the neurologist and not believing his diagnosis or prognosis. Why must he challenge everything? He didn't bring it up again, however, perhaps not wanting to tamp down the relief I felt from hearing that she would be fine by the time she was in kindergarten.

That night I did as much research as I could on cerebral palsy. I read the stats, the symptoms, the treatments and the varying degrees of the disease. Although I couldn't find one example of a child who "outgrew" it like the doctor was suggesting, I still believed him. The sadness I felt thinking Emily would have a limp the rest of her life was balanced with a strength coming over me, urging me to fight hard for her recovery. We would give her all the help she needed to overcome this.

It was Dave's day off from work and he had planned to take her to the MRI, scheduled for 3 that fall afternoon. Even with my part-time schedule, I had already burned though most of my generous amount of sick leave going to all the previous appointments. But I took the afternoon off the day of her MRI so I could be there with Dave and Emily. She was going to get anesthesia for the 45-minute scan of her brain, and that was a big deal even if the results weren't. As I was leaving the university, one of the directors asked if I was taking off for the day. I said, "Yes, Emily needs to have an MRI."

He looked at me with raised eyebrows and widened eyes. I didn't want unneeded attention. Emily's situation was minor, but the sound of an MRI on her brain made it sound bigger than it was, so I tried to dilute the importance of the appointment. I replied with reassurance, "It's OK—it's just to see if she has a mild form of cerebral palsy. She's fine!"

My brother, who lived an hour away, called that morning asking if we'd like him to come down and be with us during the MRI. I told him, truly believing that this appointment sounded like a bigger deal than it was, "No, thanks. It's not worth missing work and driving all the way down. We won't even get the results today. Besides, she's fine!"

I met Dave and Emily in the waiting room of the radiology department at Children's Hospital and, before I could get settled, a nurse called us back to the MRI area. The room had glass windows on one wall through which the radiologists and nurses would watch as Emily laid inside the tube so big it looked like it could swallow her tiny body. The radiologist explained, "Once Emily is asleep on the table, she'll slide into the machine. There will be incredibly loud noises—like jack hammers going off—while the scan takes place. That's normal. We'll put special headphones on her ears to protect her." I digested all of this while watching Dave hold our seven-month-old daughter. A nurse put an IV line in her arm and the doctor administered anesthesia causing Emily to immediately close her eyes and go to sleep.

I was unnervingly at ease with the diagnosis of cerebral palsy, so minor you'd never know, that I was able to joke with the doctors and nurses about how quickly she went to sleep with the medicine. Dave commented, "I wish we had that at home!" Our laughter and good mood continued as we waited in the chairs in the hallway during her scan. We had made it through the rough day. Per doctor's orders,

Emily wasn't allowed to eat prior to the MRI and Dave was worried that would make her miserable. But it turned out she wasn't interested in eating anyway. Instead, she took a long nap that morning before the MRI appointment.

While we were waiting in the hallway, Emily's scan still taking place, a doctor walked up to us, introducing himself as a neuro-oncologist, and asked to speak with us in the room next to where we were sitting. He wasn't the neurologist who had ordered the MRI, so I was a bit confused. Dave and I, still in our jovial spirits, smiled at each other and gave a little shrug as we stood up to follow him. The doctor walked slowly and looked ahead toward the little room we were approaching and said, "Your daughter has a brain tumor."

"No, she has cerebral palsy," I immediately responded in a very matter-of-fact tone. He must have the wrong parents. I then looked around and slowly realized that we were the only ones there. Emily was the only one in the MRI machine. Dread washed over me as I entered that small room.

The doctor pointed to the films hanging on the light display.

It was right there. Right in the middle of her brain. The size of a small orange. Anyone could see it.

Dave and I looked at each other in disbelief. He took several steps back while I stood planted in my spot, still staring at the films.

"No," I said again, then yelled, "They said it was cerebral palsy!"

I turned and looked at Dave. He stood on the other side of the small room and stretched his arms toward me. I burst into tears and walked over to him, collapsing into his arms. He held me tight as I wept. Another doctor showed up, this one a neurosurgeon. He asked, "How long has she had symptoms?"

Dave responded, me still crying into his chest, his arms still wrapped tight around me, "She's never used her right hand or drunk more than a few ounces of formula at a time. We thought she was allergic to her formula. The neurologist thought she had cerebral palsy."

The surgeon stated, "My guess is that the tumor is slow growing. It's probably been there from birth."

This whole time.

I peeled myself away from Dave's chest to look at this neurosurgeon. I couldn't believe what he just said. I could only look at him, silently absorbing that Emily had been suffering from a brain tumor for the past seven months while Dave and I screamed at each other, while the pediatrician smirked at me, while Emily cried in pain.

Both doctors escorted us out to watch as Emily was moved from the MRI room to another small room to wake up. We stood in this tiny, gray, windowless room with Emily still asleep in the hospital crib pushed up against the wall. Dave let go of me and stood over her, tears falling on her hospital gown, and whispered, "I love you so much, my sweet little pie." He appeared so broken, so defeated, so unlike I'd ever seen him. My heart suddenly broke in grief for him too.

The doctors passed us tissues and waited a few minutes for both us to regain our composure before they continued.

The neuro-oncologist said, "She needs surgery to remove as much of the tumor as possible, but we know we can't remove all of it. Given its location, it's too dangerous. Then she will most likely need chemotherapy. It all depends on what the surgeon sees during the surgery as well as what type of tumor it is."

I stood at attention, listening to him like I listened to my father as a little girl. I tried to appear brave and strong, wanting to be those things in front of the doctor. I concentrated on making my tears stop. The energy it took for me to stop my crying, though, caused me to only listen to some of the words he was telling us; I wasn't able to fully pay attention.

The surgeon continued with a warning. "If it looks too bad when I'm in there, if the damage is too significant, I will just close her up and not continue the surgery. She will likely pass within a few weeks if that's the case." He paused before adding, "We're hopeful that won't happen, but it's important that you're prepared for all scenarios."

I glanced at Dave. He took my hand. My life was breaking down, but I felt I had to keep it together in front of these strangers. A social worker now joined the group telling me my child had a grave illness. I finally turned numb and only then I was able to pay attention as more information came at us. There just wasn't time to collapse.

They took us upstairs to the empty oncology clinic, closed

because it was 6:30 p.m.—four hours after we first arrived in the hospital for the MRI. The neuro-oncologist gave Emily, who was still sleeping, a dose of steroids to ease her pain. He then told us to come back the next day for Emily to have an MRI of her spine to see if there were more tumors.

⇒ 2 ⇐

The Aftermath

Our phone was ringing when we walked in the door that night after hearing Emily's diagnosis. The answering machine picked up. It was the pediatrician. I picked up the phone as he said that he got the news. "I just heard. I'm sorry. Do you have family in the area?"

"No, they're in Connecticut."

He said, "You should see if they'll come out. It's going to be a long road."

For the first time, he was right. And with that, I hung up on him, slamming the phone down. "*Shit! Shit!*" I screamed into the air with a burst of terrified anger I didn't know I was holding inside.

I wanted to call my mom. There was nothing I wanted more than the comforting reassurance of her voice. But I couldn't do it. Four years earlier, my mom stood in the driveway and cried as she told me to have the best adventure while Dave and I loaded up the U–Haul to head to Colorado. She beamed with pride when my oldest brother left for college in a different state, then cried after the door shut, with my father hugging her, saying, "There, there." When my brother, Jeff, announced that he was going to travel the world, she told him to be safe and gave him calling cards to stay in touch and let her know of his progress, while my dad pulled out a world map to keep track of his travels. Growing up, we had home-cooked meals every night with easy banter at the dinner table. We talked about current events (my dad watched the news like most other dads watch sporting events) and my parents were always inquisitive of the goings-on of my day. How could I inflict pain on these people who loved and supported me and my brothers so much? But I knew my mom and dad were waiting for me to call with the news of Emily's MRI.

I waited until I called everyone else who knew that Emily had an MRI that day before calling my parents. They were my last call. I stoically told my dad that Emily had a brain tumor. He told me how sorry he was, asked some questions, then wanted to make sure that I told my brothers. He then handed the phone to my mom. And after I blurted out the news through hiccups and sobs to my mom, finally letting my emotions out, she gasped and said she was flying out to Colorado the next day. I got off the phone with her, just a few short minutes later, and collapsed into bed.

Dave went to the gym to try to work out and mostly get out of the house. He came home shortly after, saying he got there but couldn't do anything. He just sat on a bench, white with anger at the pediatrician who downplayed Emily's symptoms, and grappled with the horrible feeling that came with the reality that he was the one who took charge and fixed everything and now couldn't do anything. Couldn't even fix his own daughter. Neither one of us slept that night. We laid in bed in silence as the dark thoughts rattled our brains. Of course, that was also the first night Emily slept through the night. She was still feeling the effects of the anesthesia.

The next day, Thursday, we went back to the radiology department for another MRI, this time of Emily's spine. Our good mood in the hallway the day before was replaced with quiet gloominess. After the scan, we navigated in a fog up to the oncology clinic for our appointment. As we sat in the waiting room, I looked around at the people surrounding me. Babies, toddlers, and teens were sitting with a parent or two and sometimes a sibling. These kids—bald, skinny and with puffy faces—had cancer. And I realized this was going to be my new normal. These faces that I would occasionally notice and look away from, with just a quick thought of sympathy, would now be me and my little family.

The doctor called us back to an examining room and quickly let us know there were no other tumors found; the cancer had not spread. He examined Emily and explained, "Her painfully high-pitched cry is called a 'neuro-cry' and due to the pressure she felt from the tumor growing in her head. She didn't eat because she was nauseous. And she didn't use her right side because the tumor had damaged the area of the brain that controlled those movements."

The guilt came at me in a flash. How long she had suffered, and we had sat by, clueless.

"We brought all of this up with the pediatrician. How come he didn't catch this?" Dave asked.

"A brain tumor is very difficult to diagnose. The odds of someone having one are incredibly low; most doctors don't come across it. Plus, the symptoms mock other diseases." He then went on to explain, changing the course of the conversation, "It is likely she won't regain use of her right arm or leg—the damage to her brain has already been done, but with enough therapy, she may be able to gain some strength." He fed us information now, just bits at a time. Or maybe that's all I could absorb that day. The doctor gave Emily more medicine to control her pain and gave us phone numbers to call if anything should change with her mood. He bid us farewell saying he would see us again on Monday when Emily was scheduled for surgery. The neuro-oncologist was compassionate and soft-spoken, but more than that, when he looked at Emily, it was with an easy gentleness and a smile on his face. I immediately felt comfortable in his presence.

That evening the phone calls were easier as we had good news to share. *The tumor did not spread to her spine!* I would repeat over and over again to each person I had called the night before. I started to localize the pain of this horrible brain tumor and grasp at any bits of good news. I glossed over the reality of being in the oncology clinic and the fact that Em would most likely never have use of her right hand or leg. I didn't want anyone else to feel the horror I was feeling. I also didn't want any more pity or sympathy. The attention was making me uncomfortable.

Dave and I sat together on our family room couch that night after Emily easily went to sleep, another dose of steroids in her system. Dave announced, like an epiphany, "I'm only going to think positively from this point forward."

Up until this point he hadn't been talking. He didn't even call home to his parents, which wasn't all that surprising—he took off for college and barely looked back. But more alarming was that he wouldn't call his close friends from college. Instead, I was the one to make the phone calls, to relay the news, and to say, "No, I'm sorry. He just can't talk right now. He'll call you when he's ready." *Why?* I'd plead with him, not understanding. And he would just tell me it hurt too much. Dave is very talkative. I depended on him, in fact, to do most of the talking in our relationship. He is always quick with commentary or a sarcastic remark, and he has a biting sense of humor. He has a reaction to everything—good, bad, or indifferent—and he isn't likely to keep his opinions to himself. The silence from him was making me nervous.

So when he told me he was only going to have positive thoughts, I knew he had turned a corner. I agreed to only think positively with him. I was tired and I was sick of crying. With this new attitude, turned on like a switch, we watched *Friends* on TV. Like the rest of America on that Thursday night, we laughed as Chandler gave a sarcastic remark and Monica and Rachel rolled their eyes. We actually *laughed*. And it felt amazing. Doing something normal during this day of absolute abnormality turned out to be the best medicine for us.

On Friday, we met with the surgeon. He explained, "Emily is going to have surgery on Monday morning to remove as much of the tumor as I can get without damaging her brain. I'll make an incision on her scalp at the top of her ear and it will curve to the top of her forehead. It will look like a 'C' and then I'll use whatever tool is necessary to remove the tumor. The incision will be closed with staples that will need to be removed when she's healed. The operation will last anywhere from seven to ten hours depending on what I encounter." It was very surreal to listen to someone casually say they were going to make an incision in my baby's head. More surreal that I was giving this stranger permission to do so.

He went over the risks of the surgery like someone would go over a grocery shopping list. *Her vision might be affected because the tumor is near her optic nerve. She might become more paralyzed. She might have a stroke.* And I listened to him with my young, innocent optimism, without blinking or shedding a tear. He was cocky and confident when he spoke, and I loved that about him. I didn't want any sugar coating and I wanted someone who knew what they were doing to be conducting her surgery. Dave and I left that consultation feeling ready for Emily to get better.

As promised, my mom flew in that day and stayed with my brother, Mike, and his family. Dave and I wanted to only concentrate on Emily, and, frankly, we didn't have the energy to face other people. But I welcomed the sight of my family when they visited on Saturday and Sunday. By now, Emily was feeling more comfortable because she was still taking steroids to help with the pressure. However, she was very sleepy and could barely stay awake or take a feeding. Fear gripped us all. Fear about the impending surgery, but now fear that she wouldn't make it to Monday to have the surgery. She slept, again, through the night on Sunday, barely conscious now.

We sat in a busy waiting room at Children's Hospital at 6 a.m. on Monday morning with Emily still buckled in her car seat carrier and sound asleep. My knees were shaking as I watched the surgeon walk through the room toward us holding a cup of coffee and giving us a smile. I spent the night saying silent prayers for not only Emily, but also for this man. *Please, dear God, let him get a good night's rest. Let him be successful in his surgery.* And now, I added a quick plea, *Please, let that be just enough coffee to make him alert but not too much that his hands shake.*

I couldn't stop the tears from forming this time as he went over the consent forms, again stating the risks of the surgery. Then, way too fast, he said, "Okay, cover her with kisses—it's time."

I kissed Emily and he took her back to the operating room. That was it. He carried my baby to the operating room, and I didn't know if I would ever see her again or, if I did, what condition she would be in. Would she be able to see? Would she be forever paralyzed? Would he just stop the surgery because it was too late?

With a bright red face now wet with tears, I ran out of the waiting room to the restroom across the hall. I couldn't contain the hysteria of that moment and burst out with sobs I didn't think would ever end. I let myself cry while other women were coming in and out of the restroom. All were ignoring me and letting me cry my cry. I'm sure that some of these women knew how I felt and understood why I was sobbing. Here, at the hospital, I was not alone.

There was another person who understood everything I was going through at that moment: my husband. We leaned on each other throughout countless moments like this during Emily's life knowing that the other completely and fully understood every emotion one of us was feeling. I was Emily's parent just as much as he was Emily's parent. When I was feeling fearful, he was also feeling fearful.

When I was sad, he was also sad. When I had moments of relief, he also felt relief. We were one. That also meant that we were broken at the same times. We were drained at the same times. It's difficult to lean on someone who also needs someone to lean on.

My family arrived at the hospital to wait with us, and a short time later, our closest friends Steve and Sonja—they themselves with a baby the same age as Emily—arrived to wait as well. Dave met Steve at work and they immediately hit it off—two New England natives living in Colorado. I met them at the wedding of one of Dave and Steve's colleagues. When the pastor officiating the wedding recited in the vows that the wife would obey her new husband, both Sonja and I snorted. We made eye contact across the pews, chuckled, and became instant friends. Now we sat in a big waiting room and made small talk, waiting for the phone call that came each hour from the operating room. *They started; she's doing great. They are still working; she's doing great. They've taken some biopsies; she's doing great.* One hour, two hours, three hours....

At the fourth hour the oncologist walked in and sat next to me. He said, "I just came from the operating room. It looks like the tumor is slow growing and a low-grade type that will respond well to treatment. Of course, we need to wait for the biopsy results to make sure, and that takes several days, but this is good news."

I couldn't help but smile and let out a huge sigh of relief at this incredible news. A new feeling of confidence that we could get through this came through me at that moment. Dave must have felt the same because he and Steve announced that they were going to go to the cafeteria to eat—something we hadn't done in four days.

The surgery lasted seven hours. Tears pooled in my eyes when the surgeon finally came out to the waiting room, announcing, "She did great! I got a lot of the tumor removed." The relief was quickly replaced, though, by the reality of what might be ahead of us. Fear that she may have lost functioning, fear as to what she would look like, fear of the pain she might be in ... it was too much to think about. Dave and I sat stoically as we waited and waited for the nurse to bring us to the ICU.

Wash your hands. Only two visitors at a time. I was listening to the rules of the ICU as the nurse led me to Emily's bed. The ICU was a large, open room filled with roughly 15 beds, each with a wooden rocking chair next to it. Only a curtain separated the patients and their families from each other. The room was bright and buzzing with activity from dozens of nurses and doctors hovering around the beds. The beeping of the machines was deafening as we entered the room, but after some time, we almost didn't hear it anymore.

We finally got to Emily's bed. She had a turban made of bandages around her head, a breathing tube in her mouth, an IV in each arm, a blood pressure cuff on her leg, and lines attached to her chest. She was awake but couldn't cry or make noise because of the breathing tube. Her bright blue eyes locked with mine and all I could do was stroke her cheek and tell her I loved her and that everything was going to be okay. *Please, dear God, let everything be okay.*

We all took turns seeing Emily throughout the rest of the evening, never leaving her alone. Another rule of the ICU—visitors must be awake; you cannot sleep in the bedside chair. This meant I soon had to leave her side as I couldn't stay awake much longer. But I lived 40 minutes away from the hospital and couldn't fathom being that far from her. A nurse told us about Ronald McDonald House rooms available within the hospital for parents to use for the night. It was a first come, first serve basis so I quickly found them and signed myself up for a room. Dave, however, went home to sleep, shower, and make more phone calls.

That night, slightly intoxicated from the NyQuil I took to quell my sore throat and cough that had developed over the last few days, I drifted in and out of sleep. I slept for 45 minutes at a time and finally gave up on real sleep at 4:30 a.m. The room was the size of a closet with no windows, occupied only by a chair that converted to a twin bed. I had a hospital pillow and blanket with me and none of the comforts of home. It didn't matter. I just wanted to be close to Emily.

Emily remained in the ICU for one more night. My father did everything, including begging, to get me to go home for sleep that night. "Amy, you won't be able care for her if you're sick. Please. Just go home and rest." By now he was almost as worried for my health as he was for Emily's. I had admitted to him over the phone, during one of our regular updates to him on Emily's progress, that I had a terrible cough and sore throat. I finally relented and went home for sleep. But the guilt of being away from Emily that night ate at me like nothing I had ever felt before. Something primal came over me; I didn't want to leave my wounded child. My mom would often refer to me as a mother lioness not wanting to leave her cub. But it was stronger than a want; it was a need. This feeling would continue to creep over me any time Emily was sick. I crashed hard that night after a long shower and was back in the ICU by 5:30 a.m.

Emily, now propped up and breathing without the aid of a machine, was then moved from the ICU to a room on the fifth floor of the hospital that had four beds and a nursing station in it. This was a step-down room. In the ICU, Emily always had a nurse by her side. In this room, the nurse was close by, but had other patients to tend to in addition to Emily. During our stay, however, there was just one other patient in the room—another baby. The other difference between this room and the ICU was that I could sleep in the reclining chair next to Emily's bed.

That night I was filled with relief that I wouldn't have to leave Emily's side again. However, my cough was still lingering. I coughed all night long and added the stress of disturbing the other family in the room to all my other stresses. The other mom never complained, though. She, I'm sure, like me, had so much more to be worried about than a less than quiet night. Perhaps she, too, was just grateful to be next to her baby.

The next day Dave and I took time to eat in the cafeteria while my family stayed by Emily's bed. It was there in the cafeteria that the pediatrician, the one who said that Emily was stubborn and alluded to my paranoia as a first-time mother, came over to our table to talk to us. I'm not exactly sure of all he said to us due to either my lessened state of consciousness—lack of sleep, still taking NyQuil, first time eating in days—or my view of him as Enemy Number One. I just remember that he quickly left the table. Dave later told me he told him to leave. I wasn't sure what was said between the two and I didn't care to ask…. I was just glad he was gone. It goes without saying that we switched pediatricians after Emily's diagnosis.

Later that day we moved to a regular inpatient room on the fifth floor. This was the floor for the neuro patients, including oncology patients. I didn't know it at the time, but we would become intimately familiar with many of the rooms on this floor over the course of Emily's childhood. During this stay, Emily had a private room and laughed, sang, drank her formula and ate her snacks. That's right, laughed, sang and drank her formula and ate her snacks. By the time she settled into this room, she was a new baby—a *happy* baby. This child, who just weeks earlier would scream for hours at a time at a pitch we were certain was sterilizing all the men in a two-mile radius, barely let out a mew. Instead, she played with toys we laid out in front of her. She smiled at us. She drank from her bottle. Ah, we finally got it. This was the baby that all the books talked about!

I was able to stay with her during her four-day stay in this room, sleeping on the small cushion under the window. I put hospital sheets down and used a hospital blanket and pillow to sleep on this five-foot-long "bed," finally a reason to be thankful for my short, not quite 5'2" frame. There was no need for me to go home and be away from her. I used the hallway restroom to brush my teeth and used the showers in the Ronald McDonald parent common rooms when I could sneak away. Dave spent every day with us and drove home each night. My mom, still staying with my brother and his family, visited every day with my brother, Mike, and sister-in-law, Kim. Before we knew it, the surgeon said she was well enough to go home.

During the hospital stay the neuro-oncologist explained that the tumor was, indeed, an Astrocytoma, Grade I tumor. Just what he thought it was when he visited the operating room. Cancers are rated on a I to IV scale, I being benign and IV being malignant. Type I tumors usually remain benign, whereas Type II tumors can change to malignant tumors over time. Benign tumors tend to grow and push what's around them out of the way, while malignant tumors spread and destroy the cells and tissues around them. Since there is no room to push tissues around in the brain without causing damage, benign tumors located in the brain are also considered to be dangerous. Emily's type of tumor was thought to be easily treatable with chemotherapy and had a great survival rate of more than 90 percent. But, the oncologist warned, even if the chemotherapy worked now, we'd need to be careful to watch for a recurrence in the next five years and again in her teen years. This was my introduction to the not-so-fun world of medical statistics. Little did we know at the time, Emily had a knack for falling into the 1 to 2 percent chance of most stats cited to us.

The doctor also explained that it was not a genetically caused tumor, meaning that it was from the environment. With this information, I couldn't help but retrace all my steps during the nine months of my pregnancy (during which I was incredibly healthy) trying to find what could have caused that one mutated cell to develop. No clear answer formed, and we probably will never know what caused her cancer. Over time, I stopped fretting over what may have caused the tumor. It felt like wasted energy. Or, rather, it used energy I no longer had.

⇛ 3 ⇚

Our New Normal

We barely had time to enjoy our new daughter who finally smiled and laughed with ease before having to start chemotherapy. Just a few short weeks after Emily recovered from surgery, the neuro-oncologist told us that Emily would need to come into the hospital every week for a four-hour-long infusion of chemotherapy for the next 15 months. My first thought was to do the mental calculation, concluding that Emily would be two years old when chemotherapy ended, which, in turn, made me want to throw up. More than an entire year of her young life would be spent going to the hospital to receive nausea-inducing medicine. Not only did I not know how she was going to handle those appointments, I didn't know how *we* were going to manage these appointments. After all, we had just settled back into a routine, including going back to work, after being off for several weeks since her diagnosis. Perhaps in self-preservation mode, I decided to concentrate only on today and the next day. I didn't have the mental strength to think past that. This was the beginning of not looking ahead. The future had too many unknowns, too many dark threats.

My every Wednesday afternoon for the next year was spent in the oncology infusion room at the Children's Hospital, a far cry from my comfortable office at the university where I had usually spent my afternoons. It was here where Emily would receive the toxic medicine—so toxic nurses had to wear gloves and gowns while administering it—that would make her tumor shrink. This medicine would also cause severe constipation. We were warned by the doctors and nurses that it was going to be a big issue (a side effect from the chemo), but really? If that's all we had to worry about, we'd take it. The chemo

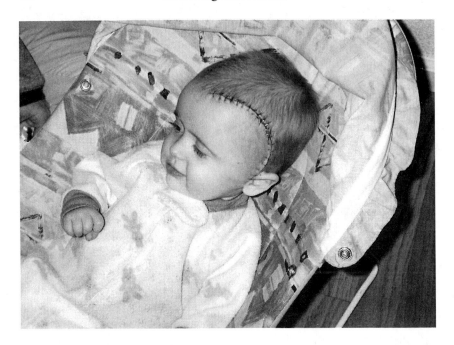

Emily after her first surgery.

would also make her somewhat nauseous and not hungry. I was used to that. Emily was always a finicky eater and skinny, not one of those babies with chunks on their thighs. And she was already bald, so I didn't need to worry about her hair falling out. My concern was occupying a one-year-old for four hours while hooked up to an IV pump each week.

Emily's first day of chemotherapy started with an outpatient surgery to implant a Broviac in her chest. This was a permanent IV line attached to a large vein in her chest that went straight to her heart. The tubing would hang outside of her chest and be clamped shut when not in use. Dave and I were quickly trained on how to flush and clean her Broviac (all the while I worried how on earth I was going to remember each step) and then sent to the oncology infusion clinic, where we sat in a little room with glass walls, feeling like aliens visiting another planet. We watched the nurses and other patients in their glass-walled rooms with intrigue as we waited for the treatment to start. Emily, meanwhile, sat on my lap and watched cartoons play on the TV hanging from the ceiling in the corner of the room. After several minutes, a cheery nurse popped in, wearing a paper gown from head to toe, and after greeting us, attached an IV line to Emily's new Broviac and pushed several buttons on the pump attached. That was it. I'm not sure what I was expecting, maybe a bang on a gong to signal the start, but certainly not the mundaneness of pushing buttons on an IV pump. The nurse floated in and out of our room for the next three and a half hours while we entertained Emily, who remained surprisingly content the entire time we were there. At the last beep of the IV pump the nurse detached Emily and we said our goodbyes until next week. No bang on the gong then, either.

Emily was a mellow, happy baby now (quite the contrast to just a few months ago). I needn't have worried too much about keeping her busy during these four-hour weekly appointments. She was so happy, in fact, that she became known as the "Dancing Queen" by the staff in the clinic. Dave, back to his slightly obnoxious, gregarious self, would stroll into the oncology clinic every Wednesday and stand Emily up on the nurses' station counter for the staff to ooh and aah

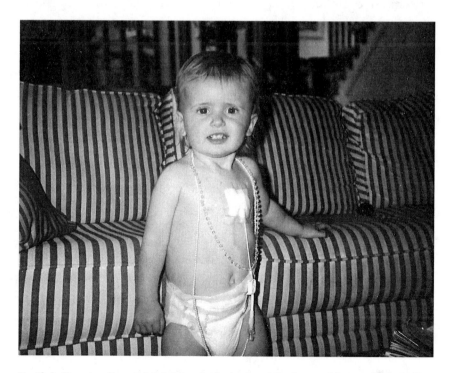

Emily's Broviac line, which blended nicely with the necklaces she loved to wear.

over her while she waited to get hooked up to the IV machine. One of the first times he did this, Emily started bouncing up and down and nodding her head to the music playing in the background resulting in the nurses joining along with her. Pretty soon, the Wednesday afternoon chemo sessions turned into festive dance parties—the nurses making sure music was playing loudly for Emily's appointments. And the staff welcomed me and Dave each week like old friends, slowly making us feel less like aliens and more like we belonged.

Week after week, we saw the same patients and their families at the oncology clinic. There was often another little girl, one year older than Emily, who was receiving her treatment at the same time as Emily. We would wave and smile and sometimes bring the girls next to each other so that they could play side by side for a few minutes. But Maria was often upset and even crying during her chemo sessions—whereas Emily would smile and charm the nurses with her dance moves. I couldn't help but be curious as to Maria's diagnosis. We couldn't talk directly because the family was Spanish speaking (and I am not), so I ended up asking our oncologist one afternoon, "Is Maria's brain tumor like Emily's?"

"Yes, she has the same type of tumor, but it's more involved in her optic nerve area and she has some issues with her vision," he replied.

Then I noticed that Maria was not in the clinic for several weeks in a row. I asked the doctor again about her. "Did Maria finish her treatment? I haven't seen her in a while."

He relayed, "No, she was having an awful time with the side effects of chemotherapy. Her parents made the decision to stop treatment."

"Does that mean…?" I started to ask. He nodded, understanding, not making me finish the question.

I paused, not able to imagine making that decision, and I grieved for those parents who had to do so. Of course, at the time, I did not know that one day Dave and I would be forced to make the same type of decision.

I cried when I told Dave about Maria. I said a silent prayer for her and her family that night and many nights after, never forgetting the little girl so like Emily.

Labs would be drawn frequently during chemotherapy sessions.

The medicine does not discriminate as to what cells it destroys, often killing the cells that help a person fight off infections on their own. Every so often during Emily's time receiving chemo, we would receive a phone call letting us know that Emily's blood counts were too low for her to be out in public. So those weeks we wouldn't take her to the grocery store or mall, and we wouldn't allow playdates. Sometimes they'd dip too low for her to even receive chemotherapy and we would happily skip the Wednesday routine that week.

During one of Emily's early chemotherapy visits, the nurse practitioner noticed her head looked slightly larger. "How has Emily been feeling?" she asked.

"Just a little fussier than normal. And not sleeping through the night again," I responded, thinking back and realizing that, yes, we had slipped into that pattern again.

She took out her measuring tape, and sure enough, Emily's head was larger than her last measurement.

"Hmm, I bet fluid isn't draining properly and is collecting in her head," she announced. "Let me go talk with the doctor." *What?* I sat nervously in the room looking at Emily waiting for the nurse practitioner to come back and say, *Never mind—she's fine.* Seriously, let's get on with our dance party.

Instead, a few phone calls later, Emily had a CT scan of her brain. It showed, as the nurse practitioner thought, Emily was suffering from hydrocephalus. The tumor was blocking the left ventricle from properly draining the fluid in her head, causing the fluid to build up. No wonder she was crying more than usual over the last few weeks. Her head was swelling like a balloon.

Surgery was quickly scheduled for her to have a VP shunt permanently placed in her brain to help drain the fluid. It was a common surgery and wasn't going to be nearly as involved as the surgery she had just three months ago. I accepted this news quickly and was anxious for her to have it placed. I wanted her pain to go away, easily discounting the threat another brain surgery posed.

I was somehow able to take more time off work (the university gave an astronomical amount of sick leave) and, thankfully, the surgery was scheduled for Dave's day off since he had no more sick or vacation days left to take. We only anticipated one night in the hospital and we were feeling ready. The phone calls were made to family and friends letting them know of the surgery and also letting them know we've got this. No need to take time off to be with us, no need to fly out, this was going to be a breeze. After all, it was a common surgery and only a few hours long.

And surgery did go as planned and the shunt was placed with no issue. As we found out throughout most of Emily's childhood, though, good news tended to come with bad news. Emily was nauseous. Not your typical upset stomach, but projectile vomiting. On me. Time after time. I had to change my clothes so often during her recovery that I ran out and had to use the washing machines at the hospital. After doing more scans to find out why she was so sick, the doctor stated she just had air pockets in her skull causing the nausea. There was nothing to do but wait for her body to absorb it.

The one night in the hospital turned into four nights and I was miserable. I slept on a two-inch-thick mattress with constant interruptions through the night, only able to eat when Emily was feeling well enough for me to run to the cafeteria. My loneliness, and resulting crankiness, spiraled out of control. Dave had to work, and the closest family members we had were Mike and Kim, who lived an hour away and were juggling their jobs and children.

Dave and I didn't go out anymore. We didn't have a babysitter. Could you imagine telling a teenager, "The baby is on chemotherapy and susceptible to basic illnesses, so you have to be 100% healthy when you come over. She has a tube sticking out of her chest—make sure she doesn't tug at it. And she could get cranky at times most likely because she's nauseous. Good luck!" Besides, we were either working on opposite days, tired, or at a doctor's appointment. Months went by without us realizing that we hadn't had a date or even an hour or two to ourselves. But beyond making time for ourselves, there wasn't time or energy to cultivate friendships that others seemed to have. I didn't feel like I had the kind of friend you could call and say, "Hey, I'm slowly losing my mind in this awful hospital room. Can you come by to gossip and talk to me about what's going on in the world?"

On the third night of our stay I overhead one of the nurses chatting with another patient's parent in the hallway. The nurse asked the parent, "Are you actually going home for the night?" The mom replied gleefully, "I am! After 30 nights in the hospital, he finally asked if Dad would come in and spend the night with him!" Thirty days. Three-zero. I told myself to shut up. I had nothing to complain about.

Once Emily recovered from the surgery, she was back to being a happy, typical baby and we fell into a routine. Every Wednesday Dave would take her to the hospital for her chemotherapy appointment and I would leave early from work to meet them there. After an hour or so, Dave would leave Em and me to finish the appointment while he went home where he would catch up on sleep or mow the lawn or go grocery shopping. Because, of course, the world was still spinning and we had to live our regular lives too.

Our new normal also included managing the Broviac line in her chest. We had to flush it nightly with Heparin, clean it, and change the bandage every three days, all the while keeping on top of the supplies needed to manage it. And now Emily had weekly appointments with physical and occupational therapists so that she could learn to use her right side. I started working a few days of my part-time job from home just so I could juggle the physical and occupational therapy visits that I insisted on going to with Emily. I quickly realized that I wanted to hear firsthand what any doctor or therapist said during her appointments. Peppering Dave with question after question on the times he took her to an appointment without me, annoying him to the point that he gladly let me handle most of them.

Typical childcare centers were not an option due to Emily's medical condition and the number of doctor appointments Emily had made it almost impossible to set a regular schedule. Dave continued working in his current position which allowed for a three-day work week, passing up opportunities to work other assignments because it would have meant working more days per week. Adding to his exhaustion was that he worked *nights* on his workdays and switched to being awake during the days I worked in the office in order to take care of Emily. I would start my work week by slipping Emily into bed with Dave after he had just gone to sleep a few hours earlier to let him know he was on baby duty.

When I was at work, I learned to turn off my emotions of home life and concentrate on work (and socializing with my colleagues). I no longer got the dreaded, pit-in-my-stomach phone calls from

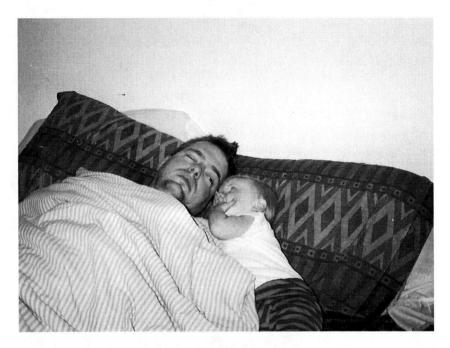

Emily blowing Dave a kiss to wake him up as I left for work. Dave worked nights and only slept for four hours before being on baby duty.

Dave saying he was frustrated with Emily and walking away. She had turned into a typical toddler. The only things now that interrupted my days at work were the unpredictable number of doctor and therapy appointments.

Thankfully, my supervisors never questioned when I would leave a voicemail saying, "There was a last-minute change in Emily's appointment this morning. I'll be in around noon." I never encountered a raised eyebrow when I said, "Emily's appointment is running late. I won't be able to make it in today after all." Instead, they adjusted my schedule whenever I needed it and gave me work I could complete at home in my own time. Caring seemed to be part of the culture, which, I later found out, wasn't the case at all places of employment. Dave's employer, also supportive but more limited due to the rigorous line of work he was in, let him attend his mandatory training days whenever he could—not the typical mandated day, which fell on Wednesday, "Chemo Day."

I didn't want to jeopardize the liberties I had at work for several reasons, the main one of which was that I needed the paycheck. We thought paying for specialized formula was expensive! We stopped buying the pricey liquid gold formula, but now paid the excessive specialist copays every week—for the oncologist, physical therapist, and occupational therapist. This was on top of all the money already spent for every other doctor, specialist, medicine, and procedure Emily had leading up to her diagnosis and throughout her treatment. But beyond a paycheck, working gave me something else to think about and the chance to be around other people, my colleagues who became my friends. It gave me a chance to escape, to do something normal.

For months and months after Emily's diagnosis, the time I spent alone with my thoughts in my 40-minute commute turned into a pity party and fear fest which resulted in sobs by the time I got to work. Thoughts of Emily's diagnosis and prognosis bounced around in my head like a wicked, ghoulish game. Once I arrived at work, I spent the first few minutes in the parking lot wiping away tears and dabbing my face with water so that I could walk into the office and pretend everything was normal. And when I got inside, it was okay, and I did feel fine. I pretended that I never had that breakdown on my morning commute—tricking both my coworkers and me. Until I broke down again the next morning.

I relished my time in the office concentrating on work, learning new things, and, most of all, chatting with coworkers. Discussing hair care products and where to get the best Thai food were some of the highlights of my workdays. This was the first job I landed after moving to Colorado. Well, actually, it was the second job. The first job I got was with a company that analyzed stocks and mutual funds, housed on the 23rd floor of a skyrise building in downtown Denver. I cried every morning going to that job, too, but only because I quickly realized that I despised corporate life. As I've mentioned, I'm quiet and soft-spoken. _Nice_ is always the word people use to describe me. That company was full of eager, ambitious people to whom I did not relate. I didn't share their enthusiasm and drive to rise to the top of some sort of corporate ladder, pushing others aside to get there. I happily quit after two weeks once I got the job offer at the university. And here, at the university, I instantly fell in step with my colleagues. They were all so _nice_. We worked on several academic research projects studying various aspects of mental health issues facing

American Indian populations. In addition to the work that was being done at the center, I loved hearing about what my coworkers were going through in their lives, whether it be an upcoming vacation, a break-up, or an adoption. These talks became especially important to me after Emily was diagnosed. Anything to take me away from my dark thoughts.

Plus, working meant we had insurance for Emily. Insurance was undoubtedly an absolute necessity that we gladly paid for each month. However, I spent a great deal of Emily's childhood fighting for basic services I thought should be included in the coverage. My first stumbling block came when the doctor recommended Emily receive weekly physical and occupational therapy and put in the referral for just that. The letter from our insurance company, though, only approved eight visits of therapy to be used within 60 days per this diagnosis. Eight visits! My now-nine-month-old baby, who was paralyzed on one side, who wasn't close to even sitting up on her own, while other babies at this age were starting to pull themselves up on furniture to walk, was to catch up to her peers with eight physical therapy sessions in the next two months (during which she was also receiving chemotherapy).

My usually calm, relaxed, quiet demeanor was brushed aside as I easily spent hours a week fighting this inane policy of our insurance. I talked with the representative, I talked with the representative's supervisor, I wrote letters to the state's insurance commissioner, I faxed documents, I cried, I made an insurance representative cry. Insurance representatives became my Enemy Number Two, a close second after our original pediatrician. Just like any mom would fight for her child's rights, I was no different. Emily needed to learn to sit, she needed to learn to walk, she needed to learn to use her hand. Physical and occupational therapists were trained to help us do just this, and we paid a lot of money each month to our insurance provider to cover such costs. In the end, my fighting worked. The insurance company changed its policy to allow 20 visits each of physical and occupational therapy *per year*.

And since the world insisted on still spinning, shortly after Emily's diagnosis, I continued with my graduate school program. I finished my classes before Emily was born and had spent the last several months before Emily's diagnosis writing my thesis. The defense, a meeting with my academic advisors to present and defend the research findings of my thesis, had been on the calendar for a while and was scheduled for the week after the initial MRI. A few days after she was diagnosed at that MRI, though, I asked to postpone this last step needed to finally earn my degree for a few months, explaining what was going on with Emily.

When that dreaded day came, I slunk into the conference room to defend a paper that, at that point, I was completely removed from. I hadn't thought of the paper since before Emily was diagnosed and I barely spent time preparing for this meeting. Three years of work to earn this degree just didn't matter to me anymore, but I was *so* close to closing this chapter of my life. So with fake confidence, as ready as I was going to be to discuss unintended pregnancy rates among certain American Indian tribes, I faced my three academic advisors. However, instead of questions on why I chose one statistical method over another or the significance of my findings, I was met with question after question regarding Emily's health, prognosis, and treatment plan. And then they congratulated me on my paper and let me go home. I had just earned a pity master's degree.

I practically skipped back to my car in the parking garage after the defense. I didn't care that I got off easy, I didn't even care that I had the degree, I was just relieved to have this behind me—it was one less thing to think about. I called my parents that night, shouting into the phone, "It's over!" They were thrilled I earned my degree. I was thrilled it was over.

Around this time, Dave and I started looking at new houses. Our crumbling starter home felt dreary while we were finally feeling like life was looking up. We saw the finish line of Emily's treatment in sight. I wasn't juggling graduate school anymore. Dave started working the day shift, finally getting some sleep. And, most of all, Emily was a happy baby now which, in turn, made us happy parents. Dave and I no longer threatened divorce. In fact, we were more of a team than ever before. And although our love ran deep, our partnership was probably due to more practical reasons—we couldn't fathom juggling all her doctor appointments and our work schedules without each other.

When Emily was 20 months old and had just a few more months of chemotherapy left, we moved into a new home on a cul-de-sac with beautiful views of the foothills. Our good luck continued, blessing us with fun next-door neighbors who were a family of three, just like us—a couple with a baby girl. Vicki was my age, easy to talk to, and didn't seem fazed by the fact that we often had appointments at a cancer clinic. Besides, we had other things to talk about—her new baby, our new houses, and other neighbors moving in—*normal* things. Her husband and Dave became friends as well, and before we knew it, all of us, including some other new neighbors, would hang out together at our house or their house on a regular basis. Of course, Emily and their baby girl would also become close friends.

When we were together, we laughed at the many moments raising a child gives that are comical (otherwise you'd cry). We'd also complain about our days at work and talk about home decorating trends we saw in a magazine. Dave and I would talk about Emily's cancer and her treatment but didn't dwell on it. We wanted to be a regular, ordinary family that fit in with our neighbors. We kept our emotions to ourselves and each other. Only occasionally did we truly open up to our new friends, but never to the depths we did with each other. Vicki and her family quickly became the type of friends who could just walk into our house, sit down, and pour themselves a cup of coffee. Life, indeed, was looking up.

Emily had an MRI of her brain done every three months since the day of her diagnosis to check the size of the tumor. These days consisted of her not being able to eat, followed by an IV placement, anesthesia, a 45-minute scan in the MRI machine, waking up from the anesthesia, juice and crackers, a visit with the doctor to get the results, and then home. The days before the MRI were filled with nervous energy, prayers, and pleas to God or whomever would listen. The evening of every MRI day was filled with phone calls to family and friends to let them know the results.

Logistically, the hardest part of the day was Emily having to fast before the scan because she received anesthesia. We had taught Emily a few basic signs from American Sign Language to use to communicate when she was a baby. My dad had read somewhere that babies can learn signs faster than speaking words and it often leads to less frustration felt by a baby so he sent us a book on the basics. Well, whoever wrote that sentiment didn't have a baby needing to adhere to fasting orders. Emily would sit under her highchair and sign the word "eat" over and over until we left for our appointment on MRI days. It would break our hearts and frustrate her to no end that we were not listening to her very clear request. It goes against any parenting instinct to *not* feed your hungry baby.

And even though we suffered with not being able to let Emily eat on MRI days, the disruption in our routine and a long day at the hospital, I looked forward to those days—probably too much. I counted down to that day and a giddy sense of nervousness would envelop me. Finally, I would know if the medicine Emily was getting pumped into her body every week was working. I would get some reassurance that the tumor was going away. It would allow me to breathe easier, at least for a few days.

MRI days also meant that I had exactly 45 minutes (the time Emily was under anesthesia getting the scan) to run to the hospital cafeteria and eat a meal without a child. And I relished this time. Often, my neighbor, Vicki, would have her mom babysit her daughter on MRI days and go with me to these day-long appointments which made me look forward to the appointment even more. We even made a rule that calories don't count on MRI days, resulting in a dessert to go with our hospital cafeteria lunch.

The first time Vicki offered to come with me to Emily's MRI, I quickly shrugged her off. She was just being polite. I thanked her and explained that it was, essentially, a day-long event filled with a lot of waiting. But she persisted, saying that she'd love to keep me company and she could get her mom to watch her baby. I couldn't believe anyone would give up an entire day to sit with me at a hospital, especially a child-free day. But she still offered, even after I pointed out all the fun stuff she could be doing instead. There was no manual on how to be a friend to someone whose child was going through cancer treatment, but if there were, Vicki could write it. We were able to gossip, complain about parenting, and talk about decorating ideas as if we were strolling through the mall instead of sitting in a room waiting for the doctor to tell me whether my daughter's brain tumor had grown. I could also tell Vicki if I was feeling nervous or had a hard morning not feeding Emily in preparation for the test. She listened to me state those things just like she listened to me when I whined about not knowing what to make for dinner. Like they were very normal things to complain about. There were no dramatics or tears and there was no handholding. I'm not the type of person who wears my emotions on my sleeve and Vicki respected that. After all, she was like that too.

Most MRI days were routine. Only two times did they not go as planned. The first one occurred when Emily was still a baby. The nurse casually mentioned that Emily developed an allergic reaction to the medicine used as the anesthesia, stating, "Emily stopped breathing and we needed to resuscitate her." She told me this after the MRI had taken place and in such a laid-back manner I just responded with an "Okay, I'll be sure to list that as an allergen on her forms." I didn't think of it again until I relayed to Dave how everything went that evening. Then, I thought, *Wait! Did she say Emily stopped breathing?* But Em was there in my arms feeling just fine at that moment. I tucked away the incident, not wanting to tarnish my upbeat mood in those days of Emily feeling good and life going as planned. Denial that Emily was up against the odds, even during routine appointments, was necessary in order for us to move on.

Later, when Emily was about two years old and just waking up from the anesthesia after a routine MRI, the radiologist informed me that they missed an image. They needed Emily go back in the machine to get that missing image, which would only take four minutes. Since she had just woken up from anesthesia, though, she would need to get the scan awake. This led to a concern from the doctors that she would get upset and move during the imagining, being the toddler she was. So the radiologist told me, "I need you to go into the machine with her. Just try to balance yourself on top of her, with your head at her chest level, and give her comfort while reminding her not to move." Essentially, I was to hold a plank for four minutes on top of her, with a gentle soothing smile on my face. Luckily my kid was proving to be tougher than me and knew to stay still since I broke my plank after 45 seconds, felt nauseous, and excused myself from the machine.

During Emily's 15 months of chemotherapy, as well as for several months after, the results and these post–MRI meetings with the doctor were great. It was easy to call home to my family and report that the tumor had shrunk again. It never disappeared during the time she was on chemo, which was the hope. But it never got bigger, which was great news.

Because of Emily's right-sided weakness (she still had no use of her right hand and limited movement in her leg) she did not reach physical milestones like typical kids. She did not sit up at six months, didn't crawl at eight months, and didn't walk at 12 months. She was also undergoing chemotherapy during much of these stages which caused fatigue and nausea. The cards were stacked against her.

We went to physical and occupational therapy religiously. It was a pain in my butt, expensive and a regular disruption to our schedule. But life would be so much easier if Emily could walk, run, and use two hands. And, eventually, with the help of this therapy, she learned to sit up. She learned to scoot everywhere by sitting on her bottom and using her left arm to drag herself where she wanted to go. Emily didn't use her right hand, but she could use it to help hold things and balance a baby doll. Those were our milestones that I boasted about to willing audiences.

I got a phone call at work from Dave when Emily was two years old. "Emily is walking!" he shouted into the phone. Emily was the apple of Dave's eye and seemed to always do something amazing to him, so I listened to this news with a grain of salt, not quite believing him. I was happily proven wrong that evening when I walked in the front door, grabbed a Hershey's Kiss from the candy dish, and watched Emily walk across the room reaching out to get the candy. She walked! She walked the length of the room! And, of course, she got the chocolate.

This was a huge deal, worthy of the excitement Dave had when he called me. I grinned at Dave who was *still* grinning. We were never sure that she would be able to accomplish this task, something most of us take for granted, and relief washed over us that she did that afternoon. The world was so much easier to navigate if you could walk. Her gait was off, and she walked with a limp, but she walked. Finally meeting this milestone, one year after most kids, emphasized the importance of going to physical and occupational therapy. These appointments took priority and we never missed a week.

Soon after we started physical therapy, the therapist suggested Emily get fitted for an ankle foot orthotic (AFO). This was a hard-plastic brace, molded for Emily's foot and leg, to help position her foot in a straight, neutral position. It would aid her walking as well as keep the foot positioned in a straight manner rather than rotating out, which it was trying to do. It was also the bane of my existence when we went shoe shopping. Trying to get shoes on a toddler is one thing, trying to get a shoe to fit over this large piece of plastic that doesn't bend is another. There was more than one occasion when I left a shoe department angry and in tears over the physical frustration and exhaustion of trying to get a shoe to fit over the AFO. I learned that I had to buy two different pairs of shoes—one in the size of Emily's left foot and the other seemingly clown-sized to fit over the AFO on her right foot. How cute a shoe was or what color it came in didn't matter anymore—the only thing that mattered was if I could get it on her foot without breaking a sweat.

Chemotherapy finally ended after Emily turned two years old and we were getting into the swing of life. We hardly had to take time off from work anymore (thanks to my part-time schedule and a few days a week at home), and Emily was healthy and catching up to those physical milestones. Cognitively, she was great. She knew all her colors, numbers and letters and loved to talk—ahead of the curve for a two-year-old. Pretty amazing for a two-year-old that had brain surgery and more than a year of chemotherapy! She was outgoing, enjoyed a good joke, and loved playing with friends as well as her cousins who doted on her. Parenting this now "healthy" baby became what we thought was normal and we breathed easier. Much easier. My relationship with Dave felt solid. We laughed again, both together and with our new set of friends in our neighborhood.

Life became so manageable once chemo ended, I added an exercise routine to my day. We lived in Colorado, consistently rated one of the fittest states, surrounded by people who were active—biking, hiking, skiing, and running—and I decided to give jogging a try. I'm not exactly sure what I was thinking as I was also the same person who played softball as a kid because it was the sport that had the least amount of running involved. But people would talk of their runner's high and how great they felt. They were also skinny. I put two and two together—I could feel great and be skinny—and started jogging. My sister-in-law, Kim, one of those skinny runners, got me to sign up for a 10K race with her to help keep me running. I found that training for that race became a cheap way to get out of the house and get fresh air by myself. I never once felt the runner's high nor did I get skinny. I ran for 20 minutes at a time, came home, and ate chips and salsa because I deserved it. But I ran that race with Kim. When I wanted to start walking at mile five, still having more than a mile to go, Kim jogged backward in front of me to the finish line, telling me the whole time I could do it and to not stop running. I wanted to call her all sorts of names during that last mile, and plenty were running through my head, but I could barely breathe, never mind talk. She gave me the encouragement I needed to not give up, though. I finished that race and reflected on that accomplishment often when I didn't think I could handle situations I was dealt (and many were to come).

≋ 4 ≋

Another Surgery

Several months after Emily ended chemotherapy, when she was two and a half years old, a routine MRI showed that a large cyst was growing from the tumor. She had shown no symptoms leading up to this MRI. In fact, I had started to think that the MRIs occurring every three months were excessive. We had gotten into a routine with our work schedules, my little jogs, and potluck dinners at neighbors' houses. I wanted this to be behind us and just be normal. But here I was staring at an MRI film showing a giant mass where Emily's tumor should be shrinking, not quite understanding how this happened. The doctor explained at this MRI visit that she needed to have surgery, like her first surgery, to remove this large cyst from her brain. Since it was a cyst that had grown, not the tumor, there would be no chemotherapy.

Hearing the word "cyst" somehow made it feel less serious than "tumor." Even though she would need major surgery, the same surgery as her first, I didn't panic. Perhaps it was the rapid pace at which this was happening—surgery was in just two days, I didn't *feel*, I just *did*. I knew I needed to pack for a week at the hospital. I had to wrap things up at work so I could be off for a week. And I had to act like this was no big deal in front of Emily.

"This time is different, though," I explained over the phone to my brother, Jeff, who was concerned we were going through this again and living so far apart. "First, we didn't even know what type of tumor Emily had the first time around or even if the surgeon could complete the surgery. Second, we know exactly what to expect with this surgery and recovery—we didn't the first time. Third, we know that Emily sailed through the first surgery and recovery. She'll do the same with this one."

Mike and Kim were planning to be with us. My parents would fly out for the surgery as well. And we had friends now. Our neighbors at our new house were like family. I knew they, along with Steve and Sonja, would visit and check in often. Work was completely fine with me suddenly taking a week off and Dave could take a few days off as well.

The next day was spent meeting with the surgeon who reviewed what he would do during the operation. The risks were the same as the original surgery, but this time the surgeon felt more confident as he was familiar with what he was up against. Both Dave and I felt ready to go through with the seven-hour surgery scheduled for the following day.

Emily was older now, though, curious and aware of her world—like any typical toddler. We learned, through our numerous appointments at the hospital for chemotherapy, to keep the trips to the hospital light and fun. We talked about the big sleepover at the hospital. *How exciting! What fun toys do you want to pack? Won't it be great that I get to sleep in the same room as you?* The last thing we needed was for her to feel stress. The biggest thing a two-year-old should worry about is whether they get dessert. She didn't need to be any different.

We arrived at the hospital several hours before the surgery for Emily to receive IV antibiotics to eliminate the risk of her VP shunt getting infected during the surgery. By now, Emily was known as "a hard stick," with tiny veins that like to roll. After a struggle, the nurses finally found a viable spot for the IV in Emily's left arm—the only arm she had use of. To make things worse, it was held in place with a large arm shunt rendering it impossible for her to use her hand. She sat on my lap, very grumpy about having to sit for hours with no use of her hands. She repeatedly complained, wanting it taken out, and I had to repeatedly tell her that we couldn't. Mike and Kim arrived at the hospital just in time to see both of us teary, frustrated, and grumbling at each other. When Emily spotted Mike, she, with clear relief, lifted her bandaged arm and said in her sweet little voice, "Here, Uncle Mike, take it off. I'm all done." The tears when he wouldn't started all over again and poor Mike lost a few cool uncle points.

It turned out that even though she had a very similar surgery before with a good outcome, it was *not* easier to sign consent forms.

In fact, Dave and I stood in the hallway with the doctor handing me the forms to sign and I froze. I couldn't do it. I had been so busy preparing for the hospital stay I didn't have time to process what was about to happen. It suddenly hit me. I handed them to Dave and went to the restroom (again) to cry. When I came out, Dave went into the restroom after scrawling his name on the forms.

Emily was given medicine, Midazolam, to relax her as well as cause her to forget what was happening prior to going back to the operating room. This was common practice for patients they termed "frequent fliers"—kids who had multiple surgeries—ensuring she wouldn't have any memory of the operating room. Another plus, she acted goofy after getting this medicine. She sang songs and repeated, "I love you, Mommy!" with a big grin on her face after receiving her dose of this medicine. The nurses in pre-op gave me a white paper jumpsuit to put on, along with a hat to go over my hair, so that I could go with my drunken child to the operating room. Here, they would put the oxygen mask on her face and blow gas that made her sleepy into her nose. And it was here that I would somehow stop all thoughts from forming. I went into self-preservation mode. I had to, because if I thought about what would happen in that room, I would have collapsed. Once she was fully asleep, I was escorted out.

On my way to the waiting room to meet Dave, I ran into my brother. Not Mike, but Jeff—who lived in Connecticut. "*What are you doing here?!*" I yelled and then hugged him with appreciation and started crying all over again. It was hard for me to understand the value of having loved ones close by during stressful times, until they were there. I'm so pragmatic; I never wanted to put someone out just to sit next to me in a waiting room for hours. But, as I learned during these times, it wasn't just sitting. There was somehow a strength that got passed from them to me. It was them sharing in all the emotions we endured during those times that made waiting easier. Like Kim, who acted like my personal cheerleader during the 10K race. She gave me the confidence to get through that hard moment when I wanted to give up. Having my siblings and parents in that waiting room empowered me. We had a mini family reunion in the surgical waiting room of Children's Hospital while my child had major surgery. It made the time go by quickly but also made me realize how strange our new normal had become.

Emily's time in the ICU after this seven-hour surgery was like the first time. She had a turban of bandages on her head, a breathing tube in her mouth, and multiple IVs. The surgeon relayed that all went well and he was able to drain fluid from the cyst, hopeful now that it would collapse and go away. Emily was kept heavily medicated for the first 24 hours after surgery, sleeping through most of it.

Instead of going to the Ronald McDonald House room at the hospital for the night, I went home to sleep. I had learned that sleep was an invaluable commodity that was not available at the hospital. Feeling slightly better about leaving Emily while she was under one-on-one care in the ICU, under significant medications, I went home late that night.

The next morning, as I backed out of the driveway of my suburban home at 5:15 to rush back to the ICU, I noticed a helicopter hovering, literally, just feet above the roof of my house. The only thought I had of this bizarre sight was "That's weird." I then continued to the hospital to sit next to my daughter, promptly forgetting all about the helicopter. When Dave arrived at the hospital a few hours later, he told me that Vicki had called wanting to know why a helicopter had been hovering over our house for so long. Dave was in such a trance he hadn't even noticed it. We learned a little bit later (on the evening news) that there was a bear wandering our neighborhood, our yard in particular, and officials were trying to spot it. At that point we could only laugh at our joint levels of delirium. And we were thankful I wasn't mauled by a bear leaving the house that morning.

Emily spent that day in the ICU, with the breathing tube still in her mouth, heavily medicated. When I became exhausted at 10 p.m. and needed to sleep, Jeff immediately offered that I go with him to his hotel room, just a five-minute drive from the hospital. Loving the idea of a real bed and a real bathroom, complete with a shower, so close to the hospital, I gave the nurse the hotel phone number to call for when they pulled the tube or Emily woke up, expected at some point during the night. Jeff was very understanding when I walked into the room, took over the bathroom and then collapsed into bed without a word. He was very understanding when the room phone rang at 4 a.m. and I flew out the door shouting, "Everything's fine, the nurse said she's awake and asking for me!"

I rushed into the ICU 20 minutes later to find Emily tossing a teddy bear around, bottle hanging out of her mouth, humming "Twinkle, Twinkle, Little Star." I could not get over the fact that this two-and-a-half-year-old woke up with a breathing tube in her mouth and had it removed, along with some IVs, all on her own without me at her side to hold her hand. It was amazing how brave and seemingly fearless she was. So unlike me, who battled a constant barrage of irrational fears as a child.

Later that morning Emily was moved from the ICU room to the step-down room on the fifth floor, already occupied by three other families. But this time, I couldn't handle it. *NO*, rang through my head as we entered the room and I saw all the other families. Emily was older now, plus I knew more. I didn't want her around other kids crying, but mostly, I didn't like all the noise and commotion. I burst into tears when we got settled, and explained, somehow, without using words, to Dave that we just couldn't be in this room. He knew. I put my Walkman headphones on, volume up to drown out the noise of other kids crying and families talking, and sat, tears still streaming down my cheeks, on the window seat next to Emily's crib as Dave left the room. About 30 minutes later, Dave, a nurse and social worker came into the room and took us to a regular single room on the fifth floor. The social worker said to me, "I see you're upset. Can we talk?"

"No, thanks. I'm fine." Really, my two-year-old daughter just had her third major brain surgery—I think she could figure out why I was upset.

Emily was able to recover from this surgery just as quickly as she had from her first one. In fact, she was a ball of energy and all smiles. She was excited that Nana and Grandpa were there visiting her along with Uncle Jeff. She was recovering at such a fast speed this time that my brother Mike and his wife Kim were able to bring their kids to visit.

Emily's cousins, Katie and Christopher, were her favorite "big kids" who always led Emily to fits of laughter. Emily used to call Christopher, who is three years older than she is, "Honey"— how Kim usually referred to him. We would correct Emily and say, "His name is Christopher." She'd agree, saying she knew, but proceed to call him "Honey" anyway. Christopher, she knew, would always answer her calls of "Honey, want to play?" with his charming smile and a nod. Katie is seven years older than Emily, dressed in trendy, sparkly clothes, and, of course, was idolized by Emily. I believe, though, the feeling was mutual. Katie encouraged Emily's love of horses by letting Emily ride her horse, expertly holding on to Emily whose balance needed much help (I was always too scared of the giant creature to be of any assistance). It was no surprise that after a few more days in the hospital with these visitors, Emily was declared well enough to go home.

Getting home for me meant showering off the hospital gunk and loads of laundry to wipe new all the outfits worn throughout the week. It meant sleeping in a real bed, lounging on the couch in the evening, and eating whatever and whenever I wanted. It meant going back to work and regular appointments. But going home also meant that I finally had time to feel and think about the enormity of the situation we were just in. It meant throwing back a shot of NyQuil in order to sleep at night. It meant running to the toilet to vomit after dinner, my stomach suddenly not able to handle the fact that it was over and I was allowed to eat and relax again.

⇒ 5 ⇐

Summer from Hell

I didn't want to call the doctor to say that Emily had a bump on her head. She fell, banged her head on the wall, and a bump formed. These things happen to kids. This was the conversation I had with Dave, who was insistent that something was wrong, and I was insistent that he was being paranoid. We had just gotten back to a regular routine following Emily's surgery to remove the cyst just two months earlier. Emily and I spent my days home from work going to physical therapy, baking goodies, and doing laundry and other mundane household chores. I had coffee with Vicki next door regularly and took Emily to McDonald's for special treats now and then. On my workdays, I relished the challenge work gave me as much as my time with my colleagues. When Dave was home from work, he would take Emily to the park, take her out to lunch with his friends, and go grocery shopping. Dave and I rented movies on the weekends and had potluck dinners every Wednesday night with our neighbors. We were fine. There was no way something was wrong. But Dave persisted and I finally backed down, not having the energy to fight him anymore. I called the doctor and brought her in for a quick exam. I was more than happy to report to Dave, in a snide tone, "They said she has bump on her head from falling down. It should bruise and go away."

But a week later it looked the same and bruising never occurred. Dave wanted to take her in again for an exam. Still angry with Emily's first pediatrician who was entirely wrong about her diagnosis, Dave didn't want to take any more chances. I, however, resisted a second appointment, still believing that I was that paranoid first-time mom. I also didn't want anything to be wrong. I wanted to be that ostrich who put her head in the sand and didn't face the possibility that something could be amiss. In the end, though, I relented, not wanting to fight with Dave again over this. I made the phone call to the oncologist who ordered a quick CT scan be done at 9 the next morning.

That night, I put Emily down at her normal 8 o'clock bedtime and she easily fell asleep. But by 10 she had gotten up so many times we finally put her in bed with me, while Dave slept in the guest room. She continued to scream and cry and scream again. At midnight Dave came in wondering if her diaper was too tight. At 1 a.m. he came in thinking she was cold and needed socks. At 2, I started crying. At 3, I yelled at her to stop crying. At 4, Dave took her temperature. At 5, I resisted the urge to spank her. At 6, we got up and laid on the couch with the TV on just hoping and praying she would calm down. She finally fell asleep at 6:30. At 7:30, Dave woke us up to say we needed to leave soon for the CT scan.

I sat with unwashed hair, bags under my eyes, Emily on my lap eating Goldfish, in the oncology waiting room waiting to see the doctor to get the results of the scan she just had. The anger I had over this pointless appointment, still believing it was just a bump on her head from a fall, was amplified by the exhaustion of the night before. Dave sat at work, probably with a cup of coffee in his hand, I bitterly thought, while I sat in this waiting room, hungry and in dire need of caffeine after rushing out of the house with no time for coffee or breakfast. It was a full hour before the doctor popped his head into the waiting room, made eye contact with me, and signaled for me to follow him back to the private exam room. My crankiness vanished. Something was wrong. I could tell by the frown on his face.

"She has another cyst," he said. "The pressure in her brain was so bad it cracked her skull leading to the bump on her face." He paused, then added, "She probably fell because the cyst and resulting pressure upset her balance. Ironically, the fact that her skull cracked, leaking fluids out of her brain, probably saved her life. The cyst is too big to survive otherwise."

I held Emily close in my lap as I came to terms with the fact that she could have died. Her skull actually fractured from the pressure of the enlarging cyst. *I yelled at her last night.* I yelled at her because she cried in pain and I was too dense to understand. I told Dave she didn't need this appointment just so that I could save face if nothing was wrong. I looked at Emily in disbelief, wondering how much pain she must have endured over this last week. I wanted to throw up. The guilt and sadness ate at me second by second. And I let myself feel those things for only the minute I had to comprehend what the doctor just said, but then I had to listen. I had to pay attention. I had to do what he was telling me to do.

The doctor wanted to have an MRI image of it so he could come up with a treatment plan. He asked, "When was the last time she ate?"

"Twenty minutes ago, in the waiting room—she had some Goldfish."

"Okay," he replied, "the MRI will be scheduled for later today. I'll let you know exactly when after I call down, but it will be at least four hours from now since she just ate." He went on to say that that we needed to wait in the hospital as they just prescribed meds to relieve her pain and he would need to administer those.

A few minutes later the doctor came back and told me the MRI was scheduled for 6 that evening. It was 11 a.m. at that moment—just seven more hours to wait.

Emotions were swiftly set aside as survival mode kicked in. After phone calls were made to update Dave, my work, parents, and friends, we waited. When the fish tank got boring, we moved to a book. When the book was finished, we watched TV. We played games in every waiting room we could find in that hospital. At one point, a friend and coworker stopped by and gave me some candy that I ate when Emily wasn't looking. I hadn't been able to eat that afternoon, not wanting to tempt Emily by bringing her to the cafeteria, and I had left the house in such a rush the only snack with me were the Goldfish Emily had eaten in the waiting room that morning.

Finally, 6 p.m. arrived and Emily had her MRI while I inhaled food and caffeine in the cafeteria. The results of the MRI were read immediately, and the doctor decided to surgically insert a reservoir directly into the cyst-filled tumor. This was basically a tube that went from just under her scalp directly into the cyst, sitting in the middle of her brain. The oncologist would then access this reservoir to suction out the cyst fluid and then insert chemotherapy directly into the tumor every day until the cyst was drained. Additionally, she would be on another course of systemic chemotherapy, like she had initially when she was a baby, but this time once a week for only three months.

I concentrated on the fact that each treatment the oncologist wanted to do was outpatient, except for the quick surgery to have the reservoir placed in her brain. We could handle outpatient. It meant we could all sleep in our beds at night, keeping some semblance of our routine. It also meant that my work and Dave's work wouldn't be as disrupted. I didn't dwell on the fact that the reservoir treatment she was about to undergo was new and that only a handful of patients had ever gone through it. Some thoughts are conveniently swept to the side.

It was now 8 o'clock on the Wednesday night before the Fourth of July. Due to the holiday the next day, we had a difficult time scheduling the surgery to place the reservoir. The earliest we could schedule it was Monday. But we were also not certain she could wait that long. The oncologist made an appointment for Emily to come to the clinic on Friday for an exam. If the medicine kept her comfortable, surgery would be Monday as planned. If not, she would have emergency surgery on Friday.

We got home that night and Emily went right to sleep, steroids helping with her pain. I was quick to follow suit, remembering in a panic, though, as I was on my way to bed, that we were supposed to host a Fourth of July party the next day. My first thought, of course, was to cancel. But on a whim, wanting just one normal day spent like most everyone else in the United States, or more likely poor judgment from lack of sleep, Dave and I decided to go on with the party.

Emily slept through the night but was a bit cranky the morning of the Fourth, and by the afternoon, she had several major crying fits that steroids made only somewhat better. The party was in full swing by now (with a lot of pitching in from friends), but all I could think was *Emily's skull cracked from the pressure of the growing cyst inside her brain. Emily is going to have brain surgery tomorrow.* Somehow, I managed to mingle enough to make it look like I was fine, leaving the horrors of what was running through my head to myself, and Emily managed to make it through the day. Perhaps all the commotion and everyone paying attention to her gave her strength as well. It certainly helped Dave and me not have to confront our fears, and each other, about the days ahead. The distraction worked on us just like it does with a child.

We arrived at the hospital the next morning as planned. I didn't feed Emily breakfast and packed an overnight bag because I knew surgery was going to happen that day. She got up several times during the night crying and was clearly uncomfortable (this time I was much more sympathetic to the cries). The oncologist popped into the waiting room and asked how Emily was feeling. I shook my head and he disappeared into the back to, I assumed, schedule the surgery. A few minutes later he called us back to the exam room. He explained, "Surgery is scheduled for 6 tonight. That's the best we can do—the operating rooms and the neurosurgeon are booked solid all day."

"Six o'clock? Okay. That gives us time to go home for a little while, at least."

"No," he said. "I don't want you leaving the hospital. There might be a cancellation and we can get her in sooner. That also means I don't want her eating."

Jesus Christ. Another day of waiting in the hospital all day long with a child who was not allowed to eat.

At least Dave was with me this time. He stayed with her and I disappeared to the cafeteria for food and coffee. Once I was done eating, he went to eat. We also met with the anesthesiologist for the pre-op appointment spiel, which I could recite in my head at this point. And by 3 p.m., we got a call that a room on the fifth floor became available and she could start receiving her pre-op antibiotics. A pit formed in my stomach as we settled into the room. Please, I prayed, may this be the last time we have to stay the night in the hospital.

Another meeting with the surgeon at 6 p.m. and another set of consent forms to be signed. I quickly signed them with barely a tear. This was a quick surgery—only three hours long. Barely enough time to eat dinner.

Dave and I met Steve and Sonja as well as Mike and Kim—our local cheer squad—in the cafeteria for a quick bite and then we headed back to the familiar waiting room. Both Steve and Sonja and Mike and Kim somehow, without ever stating it was an issue, were able to leave work and get childcare for their kids no matter the day or time. We never asked them to come to the hospital; they just showed up. Time and time again. Of course, during those moments, I couldn't wrap my head around the effort it must have taken for them to be there for us. I was just grateful to see them.

The hallways had a different vibe at nighttime. Quieter, yet more urgent. It was an eerie feeling sitting in here, the windows showing darkness and city lights instead of the usual rays of sunshine. And just a few hours later, at 9:30 that night, the surgeon met us where we were sitting. "She did great. I got the reservoir in place and pulled fluid from the cyst. The nurse will be out shortly to bring you to the recovery room. And just a heads up—Emily is madder than hell." He was grinning and winked as he gave us that warning.

He wasn't kidding. I could hear the screaming as soon as the nurse opened the door to the recovery room. I was able to hold Emily immediately—no breathing tubes or excessive IV lines this time— but her shouts didn't end. Finally, when I told her everyone who was waiting to see her, she stopped. She immediately went into stories of swimming with Katie and Honey, splashing me in the water, and then, and then, and then ... the stories did not stop. She was still talking excitedly as the recovery room nurse wheeled the bed up to the fifth floor. Kim aptly announced, "She's baaack!"

After just one night in the hospital we were able to go home. A few days later she had a mediport placed in her chest during a quick outpatient procedure. This was a central line, like the Broviac she had when she was a baby, but completely internal. It could be accessed with a quick poke of a needle, typically after numbing cream had been placed on it. It was through the mediport that Emily would receive the systemic chemotherapy as well as give blood for labs.

Two days later, she started the new chemotherapy regime, and this time the once a week infusion only took 45 minutes. Since Chemo Day fell on Dave's day off, he handled all the visits and I stayed at work. After already doing more than a year of chemotherapy, going back for a few more months didn't seem like nearly as big a deal. Plus, I just couldn't keep taking time off.

This time around, though, Emily had hair to lose. And shortly after chemo started, I noticed the hair loss. She was sitting on the floor, playing with Vicki's daughter while I chatted with Vicki. We were both looking at the girls and all I could see were clumps of

Emily's blonde hair missing. And clumps on the floor. Her hair had been sticking to me and pillows for a few days now, but I thought it was just a few strands. Without a word or even thinking, I grabbed scissors and just started cutting her hair off. I told Emily, "I'm just giving your hair a quick trim."

Vicki added, "You are looking so pretty! Now we can see your big blue eyes!" She then took the scissors from me and fixed areas that needed it. And that was it. Vicki didn't say a word to me, and I did not say a word to her. We both pretended it was a very normal moment. I never thought of Emily's hair loss again. After everything else she had been through, this was a painless, easy side effect to handle.

A few weeks later, after Emily fully recovered from surgery, we started the daily regime with the reservoir to drain the cyst. I arrived at the oncology clinic at 6:45 a.m. for Emily to receive Midazolam (the medicine that makes you forget). She sat on my lap for 15 minutes while our neuro-oncologist discussed the process, letting the medicine take effect. "You going to be okay watching me put a syringe in her head? Look away if you aren't because I don't want you to pass out while I'm in the middle of this procedure."

"I'll be fine," I said, *Don't pass out, don't pass out, don't pass out,* chanting in my head.

Emily continued to sit in my lap while the doctor put a syringe in her skull and pulled 10 CCs of fluid from the cyst inside her brain. He then inserted a new syringe into her head, this one filled with chemotherapy. She didn't flinch and I didn't pass out.

"See you tomorrow morning," he said.

This routine continued for a week. Each day our morning started at 5:15 so that we could be on the road by 6 to make it to the hospital for 6:45. I was at work by 9:30 on my workdays and Emily was back to her routine of playing, walks to the park, and trips to the grocery store. I no longer needed NyQuil to fall asleep ... we were in "Go Mode." There were no thoughts swimming in my head. Every night, I relayed how Emily did at the appointments to Dave and he nodded, said, "That's good," and that was it—there was never anything more than that. I was on a mission to just get through this period. And, thanks to Midazolam, Emily handled the routine well, never remembering the morning before. Oh, how I wanted that medicine for myself.

Finally, the end of the week came, and we could see how much the cyst had shrunk. I excitedly sat in the hallway as Emily had an MRI after the doctor pulled fluid and inserted chemotherapy into the cyst-filled tumor. But the results showed that the cyst was filling up just as fast as he was pulling fluid. We had to go back for at least another week of this routine, and he would pull more fluid at a time. My mood quickly deflated but Go Mode clicked back on soon enough.

During the third week of this routine, the doctor had trouble pulling fluid from the cyst. He was cautiously optimistic that this meant the cyst was finally drained.

"New plan," he said with a smile. "Take tomorrow off, and then, on Thursday, come in and I'll pull and pull and pull until I've got as much as I can get out in one sitting so that it collapses. I'll order another scan after that to see how much of the cyst and tumor remain. Hopefully that will be the end of the cyst."

Wednesday felt great. It was a workday for me, and I could work the entire day in the office. And Emily had a day off from this awful routine. Just one more day to get through and this would all be behind us. But when I got home that night, Emily was pouting. Dave remarked, "She had a bad day. She's been pretty cranky, and I can't get her to eat anything."

I tried playing with her and feeding her, but she was not interested in either. Then the crying started. The uncontrollable, unstoppable cry, reminiscent of when she was a baby. After listening to it for 30 minutes, trying to convince myself it was nothing, just typical cranky kid stuff, I finally decided to shut out my fear of being considered one of *those* paranoid moms (yes, even through everything we'd been through, I could not shut off that feeling). I called the oncology clinic. I relayed to the after-hours on-call doctor, who was not our regular doctor, the situation with Emily—the reservoir, the draining, the day off from draining, she's crying and crying, and then I stopped. The on-call doctor did not understand this type of treatment and told me to give her Tylenol while she called our regular oncologist. Less than five minutes later the on-call doctor called me back and asked, "How long does it take you to drive to the Children's Hospital emergency room?"

"Forty minutes."

She said, "Leave right now. Your oncologist will meet you there."

"Is that Emily?!" The triage nurse yelled across the room as we walked through the ER doors. At my nod, he sent the patient he was in the middle of examining back to the crowded waiting room and took Emily straight to an exam room in the back. Not a good sign.

The neurosurgeon, who had done all of Emily's surgeries, was waiting for us and said, while raising a needle, "Sorry, there's no time to give her Midazolam, sit down and hold her tight. I need to drain the cyst." Emily sat on my lap, whimpered, and threw up as the doctor plunged the needle into her skull. Everything happened so fast I didn't have time to feel anything. I just sat, holding sweet, little, almost three-year-old Emily tight, and I watched as he drained more than 40 CCs of fluid directly from the cyst in her brain. The oncologist walked in, got on the phone and ordered a CT scan.

She lay on the table to get the CT scan, no longer crying, but shivering. Teeth chattering so hard I thought they were going to break. I asked for someone to bring her a blanket. Wrapped like a burrito, she had the two-minute scan of her head done. "Why is she so cold?" I asked more than once. "She just went through a fairly significant trauma," the doctor relayed. "She'll settle down once she's at home. But if she gets a fever, call me."

He went on to say, with concern lining his face, "She couldn't go the one day without getting fluid drained from the cyst. It had blown up. And even now, although the scan showed the cyst much smaller, it still had fluid in it after the surgeon just pulled 40 CCs."

"Now what? Do I bring her in tomorrow morning for the big draining?" I asked, wanting him to say yes to get this over with once and for all.

Instead, he said, "Let her recover tomorrow. It's late. She's been through a lot. He just pulled a ton of fluid. Bring her in on Friday for the big day."

We got home late that night and Emily was a new person. She was a happy, talkative girl who did not have a screaming headache. We were eventually all able to settle down and get a well-deserved good night's sleep. But the next morning, as Emily watched me get ready for work, I watched her. She moved as if in slow motion, had a flushed face and glossy eyes. I took her temperature and it was 104 degrees.

After a call to the clinic, which said to bring her in for IV antibiotics, I packed a bag full of snacks and toys for Em—by now I knew this could be a few hours. I called into work, again, and took off to the hospital. Walking down the hall, from the parking garage to the oncology clinic, I was met by both the oncologist and the surgeon. They told me she was going to get admitted for IV antibiotics and would have surgery the next day to have the reservoir removed. The cultures had come back from the fluid they pulled from the reservoir last night. It was swimming with bacteria. The reservoir inside her brain was infected.

Emily sat on my lap as they hooked up the IV and proceeded to throw up multiple times—on herself, me, and the nurse. Some anti-nausea meds administered, antibiotics started, and she was feeling better. Finally having a calm minute, I called home and talked with Dave to come up with a plan. I needed clothes to change into since I was sitting there with Emily's vomit on my jeans, causing me to get nauseous. And I needed an overnight bag since we would be here for a few days. He knew and was already packing my bag—the doctor had called to let him know the plan while I was on my way into the hospital.

Dave met me in the clinic 45 minutes later and handed me the overnight bag he packed. I quickly went to change as he sat with Emily. Moments later, as I stood in the restroom with my pants off, digging through the bag for something comfy and not covered in puke to put on, I shook my head and started laughing. There were no sweatpants or jeans or even pajama bottoms … just one pair of my good black linen dress pants, several shirts and a very complete make-up bag. _You've got to be kidding me._ Did he think I was going out on a date? Why so much make-up? And why no pajamas? It was either a laugh or cry moment and I couldn't cry anymore.

Looking fancy, we walked up to the fifth floor. I glanced at Dave and asked, "Why no sweatpants or jeans?"

He shrugged. "I thought those were sweats and I couldn't find your jeans."

I let it go; there were obviously more important things to be thinking about. I wasn't anxious as we settled into Emily's inpatient room, just happy Emily was feeling better and hopeful we'd be home in a few days. That was it. I didn't think about the big picture—what this meant as far as treating the cyst and tumor. We still only thought of today and tomorrow.

The nurse then delivered a pair of scrubs for me to wear, chuckling at my dilemma. My brother, Jeff, who was getting regular updates in Connecticut, had called the nurse's station to explain my clothing situation and asked if they could do something to help me out and avoid having Dave make another trip home in order for me to have something comfortable to sleep in.

On Friday, Emily had surgery to remove the infected reservoir. The surgery went as smoothly as it did when she had it put in. Knowing that it was just a three-hour surgery, and that the first one went well, I barely blinked when I signed consent forms. Brain surgery, it seemed, was becoming benign.

She spent the weekend in the hospital recovering from the surgery and receiving IV antibiotics. I was certain that we were going to go home on Monday which made getting through the weekend at the hospital tolerable. Besides, people were able to visit on weekends and that was always a treat for both Emily and me.

Emily wasn't quite her same spunky self yet. She still had a low temperature and was tired. But she played with toys in her crib and joked with the nurses. She would also wake easily in the middle of the night when the nursing staff took her vitals—every two hours—which meant I spent a lot of time coaxing her back to sleep. At one point I put a movie on at 2 a.m. because she wouldn't go back to sleep. This became a bit of a habit during this stay and, on top of everything else, I worried we would have serious sleep issues when we got home.

Monday morning finally arrived, and her oncologist came to the room. He leaned over Emily's crib and watched her silently for several minutes before speaking to me. "She's quite a trooper for enduring all that she has over the last few weeks." This doctor always spoke with the kindest heart. He, too, had a daughter who was close in age to Emily. I looked at him like he was a family member—someone who genuinely wanted the best for Emily and hated that sometimes it meant she had periods of feeling bad.

"Yes," I replied, "she's one of the strongest people I know." She endured it all without complaint and usually with a smile on her face. I then asked, "How much longer does she need antibiotics?" Ultimately, I just wanted to know when we could go home.

"That's not my call to make. She's a surgical patient. You'll need to talk to the surgeon."

Not much later the surgeon's entourage of residents and interns came parading into the room without the surgeon as he was in surgery that morning. I put the same question to this team after they were done examining Emily. One of the interns responded, "We're not certain, but she probably needs IV antibiotics for a few weeks."

"*What?!? Weeks?* Can't she just take oral antibiotics?"

They talked to me about it more and thought perhaps we could go home with the IV as I had experience with lines given her time with a Broviac. I realized midway through my conversation with this group, though, that they really didn't know the answers to my questions and were guessing. My experience with all the doctors and procedures up to this point gave me more confidence in my knowledge of how this worked, so I didn't spend much time dwelling on the prospect of either being in the hospital for a few more weeks *or* taking her home with an IV attached. I was going to wait to talk to the surgeon myself.

That same morning, I started to feel sorry for both myself and for Emily. She was still not her typical cheery, talkative self and still had a nagging fever. And I didn't know the plan. I hated not knowing the plan. We should be at home today. It was a workday for Dave, but Emily and I would be at home doing things like going to the park with our neighbor after the physical therapy appointment. I could brush my teeth in my own bathroom and take a shower when I woke up in the morning. I could sit on the couch with Emily while I drank coffee and read the newspaper and she watched *Clifford*. We could cook dinner together that night and greet Dave at the door when he came home from work. We could sit at the table together and talk about our day. Our regular, routine, boring, nothing-out-of-the-ordinary day.

Feeling pathetic, I pulled out the leftover chocolate cake that Kim had brought over the weekend to celebrate my birthday. I found a plastic fork at the bottom of the bag, took a rail down from Emily's crib and hopped on for an impromptu pity party. We sat together in the crib, at 9:30 that Monday morning, taking turns with the fork, eating cake right from the container. On par with my morning, five minutes later, the hospital social worker decided to visit our room on her regular rounds. Sitting inside the crib with Emily, a half-eaten chocolate cake in front of us, Emily wielding a chocolate-filled fork and me with a mouthful of cake, I greeted her with a sheepish smile. Thankfully, she just grinned and said, "It certainly looks like a good time for chocolate!" Finally, some understanding.

By Tuesday I still hadn't seen the surgeon and was growing more and more restless not understanding what the plan was for her treatment and discharge. However, mid-morning the nurse came in, stating, "Today might be the day you get to go home! I talked with the surgeon this morning and he's leaning towards letting you go home, but I'm waiting for more direction before I give you final news." Now thrilled with the idea of going home, I immediately called Dave at work to let him know. Our typical hospital routine was that I spent the nights at the hospital and he would visit on his days off. But the nights were lonely—both for him and me—and we didn't see him at all on his long workdays. He was just as excited as me to hear the news that we might be home that night.

Emily, though, started crying. Then she was screaming. I called the nurse back and asked for Tylenol. Maybe the fever was bothering her or perhaps there were air bubbles like she had with the VP shunt surgery. The nurse came in to examine Emily and then called the surgeon. Instead of Tylenol, he ordered morphine and a CT scan. And just like that, my packing stopped and we were on our way to the radiology department.

The surgeon met us back at our room after the scan and announced, "The cyst filled up again. It's huge. I need to drain it."

"How can you drain it? The reservoir is gone now."

"The hole where it was hasn't closed yet. I'm just going to go in there and drain it without the reservoir."

I thought he was joking. But, an hour later, 60 CCs of fluid lighter, Emily felt like a million bucks. She was talking, smiling, eating crackers and drinking juice.

Later in the day I had a long talk with the oncologist. It finally occurred to me that without the reservoir, there was no way to drain the cyst. I needed to understand what was happening and what her treatment plan was. "She has this cyst, growing from tumor cells, which keep filling with fluid. What can be done?" I asked.

He was very candid with me in stating, "Honestly, I'm not sure what we can do at this point. I'm talking with several doctors about options."

"What about radiation?" I asked, knowing it was a common cancer treatment.

"I strongly urge you against that right now. It would damage her functioning brain too much. There is work being done on a new radiation technique that would pinpoint the area in the brain where the tumor is, and until that happens, which hopefully is soon, I don't recommend it as a treatment for Emily."

Anxiety crept up in me with this news. I appreciated the candor, but suddenly felt hopeless. No longer was I worried about getting back to our regular, normal routine. I was scared for Emily's life. There might be no more treatment options. The reality that she was battling a deadly illness hit me in that moment like a sudden slap in the face.

I sat in the hospital room recliner next to Emily's bed wishing, at this point, that she just felt no more pain. That's all I wanted. That's all I prayed for. Thoughts of anything else vanished—not even hopes for her getting better. Just, please, no more pain. Of course, I kept my hopelessness to myself. Not even muttering my thoughts to Dave. We had made a vow to be positive.

The next day I was pacing the room anxious for rounds so that I could see the surgeon and tell him I needed them to think of something to do or to just let us go home. I became obsessed with getting us home. But, again, the surgeon didn't show up, just the interns. I called the nurse to my room and *demanded* to speak to the surgeon. She came back to the room to say he wasn't in his office that morning. I told her to find him because I needed answers. This mother lioness was on a mission.

Forty minutes later the surgeon briskly walked into the room and without a hello announced, "I met with the oncologist early this morning. We decided the best option was to do another major craniotomy to remove the cyst. I've got to be honest with you, though; I don't want to do the surgery—most kids have possibly two craniotomies max. This will be Emily's third and she's not even three years old. But it looks like it's the only option."

"Same type of surgery as the last one?"

"Yes. I'll schedule it for Friday." Sarcastically, but with a smile, he added, "Can I go back to the operating room? That's where I was when I got pulled out to urgently meet with you." I nodded my consent with a shrug of my shoulders. I didn't care that I pulled him out of surgery. This was my baby's life we were talking about. Quiet, reserved Amy was a thing of the past.

I called my parents after talking with Dave, relaying the plan. My dad suggested we do some further research on other options and to talk with our neuro-oncologist more on his thoughts regarding treatment. The gravity of the situation, and crossroads that we were at with her treatment and prognosis, was felt by all of us now.

The oncologist showed up in our room shortly after the phone calls. "What do other patients like Emily do? The surgeon didn't seem happy with the decision to go back in again," I asked.

He responded that there really were no other patients whose tumor presented like Emily's. Most kids with a cystic tumor, he explained, have a thin wall of tumor surrounding the cyst. The chemo can destroy that thin wall, or it can be completely removed with surgery. The tumor in Emily's brain had a thick wall and the cyst filled so

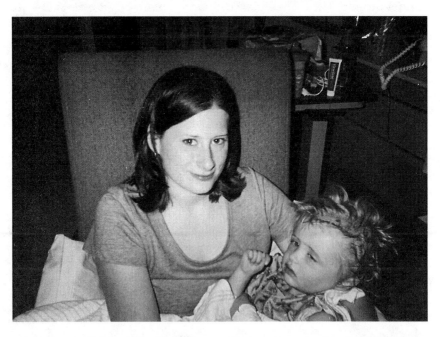

I held Emily after her third craniotomy (and sixth surgery on her brain). She was just two and a half years old.

fast it diluted the chemotherapy rendering it useless. It was also in a place where removing the whole tumor was not an option.

I knew from doing my own research that we were under the care of one of the leading pediatric neuro-oncologists in the world. He was the doctor patients were referred to from other regions. I also knew that he did his due diligence in consulting the limited number of other pediatric neuro-oncologists out there and wanted the best for Emily. Out of options, I left my trust in him.

Having this plan, albeit not a great one, focused me. I was able to concentrate on making Emily comfortable as well as rallying the troops knowing we were going to be in the hospital for at least another week as Emily recovered from yet another craniotomy. My sister-in-law, Kim, again without comment on how she was arranging childcare or rearranging her schedule, spent the night with Emily, allowing me to go home to shower, sleep, and pack for the week myself. Both she and my mom had offered to stay with Emily through the night on previous hospital stays, but I never wanted to leave Emily. This time I was spent. It was too much of a roller coaster ride. Dave felt it too and I wanted and *needed* to be with him that night. Our daughter was in dire danger and it felt like we were losing the battle.

≥ 6 ≤

And Another Surgery

During the pre-op appointment with the surgeon, Dave and I held hands as we listened to the surgeon state, "I can't keep doing this. I am going to be more aggressive than I've ever been in the past with her." He then reviewed the risk factors, patted my knee, and left the room. With scrunched up faces and tears in our eyes, we commiserated about how awful it was talking with that man. The same man who helped save our daughter's life, time and time again.

My mom flew in that night and it was 11 o'clock by the time Dave picked her up from the airport and brought her to our room to stay with us (it was a two-patient room occupied by only Emily). Dave was going to stay home until she was out of surgery for this one. He told me he could pace just as easily at home. I was at ease with this since I had my mom with me and Mike and Kim coming for the day. Plus, I felt Dave's stress. Having him at home might be easier on me. Alone, I signed the consent forms at 6 the following morning. I didn't cry. This was just one step closer to Emily getting better and us getting home.

The surgery was longer this time. Dave lasted at home for just a few hours—he was at the hospital pacing the hallways by 9:30, the urge to be close to our daughter affecting him more than he thought. The afternoon was long, and the conversations dwindled. Finally, nine hours later, the surgeon came out to meet us in the waiting room to say it was over. He drained the cyst and removed a lot of the tumor. Some pieces of tumor remained entwined in the optic nerve as well as in her brainstem—those were too dangerous to get out. He also made a last-minute decision to make a hole in one of the ventricles and connect the cyst wall to the ventricle. His hope was that if, *when*, the cyst filled again, it would fill into the ventricle which was designed to drain fluids (with the help of the VP shunt).

The surgeon patted my knee again when he was done talking and I couldn't stop the tears from pooling in my eyes and dripping down my cheeks. I was too emotional to even say thank you. I couldn't form words. I was tired. I was tired for Emily. I was tired for Dave. And I was angry Emily had been put through another surgery.

Getting to see her shortly after the talk with the surgeon did not lift our spirits like it had in the past. There she laid, the familiar turban on her head, the breathing tube in her mouth, an IV in every limb of her little body, chest monitors on, and this time a tube up her nose through which she was vomiting. The vomit was happening at a constant rate and she was thrashing her legs.

"What's happening?" I frightfully pleaded to the nurse standing over her. I was interrupted, though, by the surgeon who suddenly appeared in the ICU. From the doorway he shouted to our nurse, "Is she moving both of her legs?"

"Yes!" the nurse yelled back at him.

"And the arms? The right one?"

"Yes," responded the nurse.

As he made it to Emily's bedside, examining her himself, he said to Dave and me with a huge grin, "I didn't knock her all the way out so that I could check her movements. I needed to make sure she wasn't paralyzed. The decision to connect the cyst to the ventricle was incredibly risky. Look at her, though—she's doing great!"

With that he upped the morphine. But it didn't stop her from throwing up or settle her down.

"Please get her comfortable," was all I could mutter to the nurse. I wasn't feeling at all as jubilant as the surgeon. It was clear to me that Emily was in excruciating pain. After a quick X-ray they adjusted her breathing tube, but she still thrashed and threw up through the tube in her nose. This continued for more than an hour. Dave walked away, unable to watch. Mike showed up next to me and asked the nurse repeatedly to give her more morphine. My mom came after Mike and quickly left. Kim was next. She stood beside me and cried.

Finally, with enough morphine and Midazolam flowing through her veins, Emily stopped throwing up and thrashing. I sat, numb, next to her, stroking her cheek and holding her hand for the rest of the day. That night my mom and I went home and slept—Emily was still passed out from the incredible number of drugs now in her system. She continued to sleep all through the next day. I functioned in a fog during this time. I went through the motions of just sitting next to Emily and taking coffee breaks.

The breathing tube was removed on her third day in the ICU, replaced with an oxygen mask because her breaths were still too shallow. But the removal of the breathing tube meant I could hold her. I sat in the wooden rocking chair next to her bed in the ICU as the nurse placed Emily in my lap. Her bandaged head resting on my arm, her left eye swollen shut, oxygen mask on her face, IVs in all her limbs, heart monitors attached to her chest, but all I saw was perfection. I just felt grateful to hold her in my arms after watching her suffer for too long.

She was moved up to the fifth floor room that night, even though she hadn't really woken up. Her cousins came to visit that day and tried their hardest to get her to wake up. When she was awake it was for just a few minutes at a time and she was grumpy. We spent our time trying to figure out what could be causing her discomfort. Feeling defeated and unable to help her in any other way, I called for the nurse and said I needed to hold her. She disconnected a few of the monitors then placed her in my lap. My lap was all I had to give.

A few more days went by with Emily in this lethargic state. Not sitting up, not eating, and now running a low-grade fever. I dreaded the phone calls that were pouring in, wondering how the strong little trooper was doing. I could only put a positive spin on so much. *Probably just a few more days here!* I would optimistically say into the phone. *She's okay, just a little sleepy!* I didn't want to say the truth because I didn't want to make the other person upset or uncomfortable nor did I want to hear the "I'm sorry" or the pep talk that would naturally follow.

I was also in constant communication with my supervisor at work, who was also, at this point, a good friend. She kept telling me not to worry about work, which was good because work was the last thing on my mind. I'm not sure how I got so lucky to work with this group of people, but I was grateful. Dave had no leave left to take so he was working his three-day shifts and visiting us in the hospital on his days off.

I relayed to the oncologist during one of his visits to our room my concern that Emily was not bouncing back like she had in the past. He was not surprised, though, reminding me of everything she had been through over the last several weeks ... chemotherapy in her system, raging infection in her brain, major surgery. The oncologist asked me, then, about the movement in her legs. "Yes," I responded, "of course they are moving," annoyed now with this question. He reiterated how risky it was to attach the cyst to the ventricle given how close it was to the area of her brain that controlled her motor skills. The surgeon called him during surgery wanting his opinion if he should make the move. The oncologist agreed he should do it, but, of course, worried about the risk of her becoming paralyzed. "Well," I told the oncologist, "I'm glad you left me in the dark on that until you knew she was fine." I also couldn't help but wonder what this situation would feel like if that surgical move was not a success. The graveness of her health was becoming more apparent with each passing minute.

And then the oncologist told me that the tumor biopsies had come back and it was now graded a Type II tumor, instead of the Type I tumor it was initially. I filed that away, not able to comprehend any more at that time. *Please*, I silently pled, *no more news. Just let Emily get better.*

Emily was awake more and more but didn't want to move. She was most comfortable lying flat on her back. So the TV got angled to where she could see, and we would crane our necks and arrange our backs to hold books over her as we read stories while she listened without comments, smiles or giggles. Then, my mom got up in a flash and said, "I'll be right back!" Twenty minutes later she appeared with a large paper bag full of stickers. Emily loved it and she got moving. She put stickers on all her stuffed animals, her crib, and, her most favorite, Nana's face. This sparked uncontrolled giggles.

My mom left for Connecticut the next day, the same day physical and occupational therapists started working with Emily to get her sitting up and walking again. I fought the urge to yell at them to leave her alone ... hadn't she been through enough? But she needed to show the doctor she could get back to baseline in order for her to get sprung from this place, which felt more and more like prison with each passing day. I kept my eye on that prize as the therapists worked with Emily and didn't allow her to quit. That same day, she sat up in bed.

We had now been in the hospital for more than two weeks. Prior to that, we had spent every morning at the hospital getting chemotherapy injected directly into her tumor. I was scared. And I was exhausted. I missed Emily's laughter and incessant talking. I missed my husband. I missed our cat. I missed sleeping through the night. I missed eating when I got hungry. I missed having my own bathroom. I missed taking a shower when I wanted to take a shower. I often called Dave in the evenings after Emily went to sleep and just cried, him on the other end of the phone telling me it all would be okay. I stayed positive in front of Emily and most everyone else, even though it got harder and harder. I never let Emily see me cry. She needed to see strength and optimism and that's what she got. Faking it for Emily probably benefited me just as much.

Emily finally started walking during one of the physical therapy visits. It was while holding hands with a therapist and only a few steps at a time, but it was, literally, a step in the right direction. Then she ate a few French fries that same night. It was a great day, but I remained only cautiously optimistic. I had been burned too often at this point.

My prayers were finally answered. The following day we were allowed to go home. I may have lied to the doctors regarding the amount of food she ate, the amount of sitting up and playing she was doing, and the amount of walking around the room she did to grant us the discharge papers. But this also wasn't my first rodeo. I knew she was weak from everything she had been through. She would get stronger at a more rapid pace sleeping in her own bed without beeping and interruptions every few hours. Fifth floor, may I never see you again.

Emily was greeted at home by a giant dollhouse my parents sent while she was in the hospital. Dave stayed up late the night before assembling this beautiful, realistic house. She immediately walked over to it while holding my hand and started playing with all the dolls and furniture. She didn't talk, didn't smile, her sparkle diminished from that last round at the hospital. We brought a chair over for her to sit in since she could only stand for a minute or two at a time. But she played.

It took Emily another two weeks before she would start walking again on her own and another few weeks after that to get back to her baseline functioning. She also had to resume her weekly chemotherapy visits. Several times those were cancelled because her blood counts were too low to receive any more medicine. The three months of chemotherapy turned into six months with all the weeks off due to low counts.

It also took several months for me to feel like I was back to normal. The first few nights home were filled with the typical bouts of vomiting after eating and shots of NyQuil to stop the thoughts swimming in my head as I laid down to sleep at night. But this time, I wasn't overly excited. I wasn't grinning just from the fact that we were home and Emily was on the road to recovery like I had in the past. I snapped at the grocery store clerk when she was being chatty and I was trying to quickly get back home. I snapped at Dave when his friends unexpectedly stopped by to visit. I cried every time I drove to work. I avoided my friends because I just wasn't in the mood.

I made an appointment with my doctor because I also had started experiencing extreme heartburn, the chest pain keeping me up at night more than my thoughts. While giving me medicine, short term since she believed the heartburn was stress-induced, she asked about my mood in general. When I explained that I was still a bit down, she suggested an anti-depressant. "No, no," I said. "I'll get over it."

She said, "I believe you will, but why not help the symptoms until you do 'get over it'?" She prescribed an extremely low dose of anti-depressants.

I reluctantly started taking the medicine. I was ashamed and embarrassed I had to take this to cope. But something had to change because I knew that it wasn't healthy to go on in my current state. Dave was eager for me to take the pills—he was frustrated with my uncharacteristic dark mood. I thought about therapy and even made a few phone calls, but, frankly, I didn't want to juggle yet another appointment (and copay) during the week. So I took the tiny white pill every morning. And within a few weeks I noticed that I wasn't snapping at people so much, especially Dave. I found myself looking forward to a girls' night out that my friends had planned. It was actually working, or I was "getting over it." I continued the medicine for about four months and then weaned off. It helped me get over the hump of overwhelming sadness I felt for Emily and myself.

The months after this surgery also meant resuming all of Emily's regular doctor visits, now including a pediatric ophthalmologist who worked closely with our neuro-oncologist. Emily's right eye was not aligned with her left eye, a result of the surgery and/or tumor. She also had limited vision in her right eye following this last surgery. Six months after her last brain surgery, she had surgery on both eyes to correct the alignment and hopefully improve her vision. This outpatient surgery should have been easy for me to cope with but there were two issues I had to face. One, our insurance plan didn't cover this doctor, so we had to have someone new do this surgery (my fighting this did not end in victory). Two, I couldn't stomach the idea of anything to do with eyes. I could barely watch Dave put in his contacts in the morning without gagging, how on earth was I going to be able to help Emily with this? "You watched the doctor put a needle directly in her head on a daily basis and yet you are freaking out about an outpatient surgery on her eyes?" Dave could not understand that this was the line I was drawing on what I could handle. But the surgery was scheduled on Dave's workday which was my day off, so I put on my big girl panties and held her after surgery, watching blood-stained tears drop from her red eyes. I offered comfort as much as I could all the while trying to look away, suppressing the nauseating shiver in my body. Thankfully, Emily, who proved again that she was stronger than me, recovered nicely and *quickly* from this surgery without much fanfare, and her eye alignment improved drastically.

⇛ 7 ⇚

Another New Normal

I was growing tired of my long 40-minute commute and started applying for jobs closer to home. Within a few weeks, I received a call back for a position at a state agency office that was just 10 minutes from my house. It was for a part-time position, but more hours than I was currently working at the university which made me nervous. I was also terrified to leave all my friends and colleagues at the university. Those people knew me and my circumstances. I wasn't sure I was up for the challenge of meeting new people and explaining that I might have to be off for a week at a time due to some unforeseen health issue with Emily. And I didn't know if I could handle more hours given the number of PT, OT and doctor visits that Emily had on a regular basis. But the commute....

At the end of my interview I asked what the schedule would be for this position. The woman interviewing me replied, "Everyone works 8 a.m. to 5 p.m., with a one-hour lunch break. Because this job is part-time, you wouldn't have to work one afternoon a week." Nope, I quickly thought to myself. There was no way I could make that schedule work. When I got called back for a second interview, I almost declined it. It would have been a waste of time considering the schedule I needed. However, desperate to get away from my current commute and be closer to home, I decided to go. It obviously went well because at the end of the interview they offered me the job. I couldn't accept because of the schedule, so I shakily told them my circumstances as well as scheduling issues. "No problem!" the director of the agency exclaimed. "Would you be able to work from home a few days a week and work a few days in the office?" *Do ducks quack?* I accepted the job on the spot.

To say I was happy to have more time at home and less time commuting was an understatement. When I started my new job, Emily was fully recovered from her last surgeries and finished with the weekly chemo appointments. She could run, jump, talk, scream and be as silly as the next three-year-old. She was never shy and never, it seemed, stopped talking. She also started preschool with the public-school system. Our physical therapist had set this in motion when she casually mentioned during one of our sessions, as I paid the copay for that therapy visit, that we should contact the county for services. No one else had mentioned services, and besides, I was certain that Emily didn't need anything else—we had a nice home, we were able to juggle our jobs without putting her in childcare, we paid for all the visits (although we could barely pay for anything else), and we had insurance for Emily. But the therapist went on, saying, "Many kids with special needs, like Emily, are eligible for a Medicaid program."

I still wasn't sure why she would need it, though, since Emily had insurance through Dave's group policy at work. The therapist explained, "You would still keep the insurance Emily is on and just add Medicaid as a secondary insurance. Then Medicaid will pick up any of the costs of medical appointments that the primary insurance doesn't cover, like the copays." She went on further, given my hesitation, "You might be swinging it financially right now, but you need to think down the road. She is going to be going to several specialist doctors and therapists for years. And what if she ever needs equipment or braces? Medical bills add up quickly. I've seen it destroy many families."

The next day I called the phone number the physical therapist gave me to get more information—this seemed too good to be true. But they did indeed verify what the therapist told me. I started the lengthy process and several weeks later learned that Emily qualified for Medicaid. She also qualified for physical and occupational therapy visits which the public-school system would provide during preschool. I thanked that physical therapist profusely after we added up how much we were spending on medical copays.

We were so excited when we learned Emily could receive Medicaid until we got to the part of the letter which stated that there was a three-year wait list to receive this service. So we continued paying the exorbitant copays, now joking that it was like paying college tuition for a toddler. But Emily was able to start school right away and receive PT and OT there (she also continued intensive weekly PT and OT visits at the hospital).

On Emily's first day of preschool, I took the day off so both Dave and I could drop her off. She, of course, in her happy, confident nature, didn't even say goodbye to us—just walked in the door. Her blonde hair had grown back, and she wore it in a cute chin-length bob. She wore the outfit we picked out special for her first day of school, a pink skirt and matching short-sleeve shirt, and she toted a backpack on her back. The teacher greeted her with a big smile. "Hi, please hang your backpack on the hook and have a seat at the table," which she happily did. Dave and I stood at the entrance to the school, watching, not knowing what to do or where to stand.

Finally, Dave said, "That's it? We just leave her here and come back in two and half hours?"

"Yes," the teacher laughed.

The realization of what that meant for us hit us in a flash. We practically ran to our car. We proceeded to go straight to a restaurant where we had lunch, just the two of us out to eat in a place that wasn't a hospital cafeteria, and lingered over dessert *and* a daiquiri. Dave and I talked about how incredible it was to have this small break to look forward to on a regular basis. Emily had been by one of our sides every day of her life for more than three years.

Emily loved school. Rather, she loved her friends. And she had many. The kids didn't treat her differently because she only used one hand, wore a brace on her leg or walked with a limp. Besides, Emily was a happy, no-drama kid who was not hesitant to play with anyone she came across. She loved playing house and *running*. I, though, dreaded the inevitable games of tag that the kids played each afternoon waiting for the preschool doors to open. She always looked like she was one second away from wiping out, with her uneven gait and brace on her leg. "Wow," said one of the other moms, "she can really whip around!"

She was invited to many birthday parties and playdates during her preschool days. At this age, she needed the same level of supervision and assistance as other young kids. The only differences, I would explain if I dropped her off for a playdate, was that she would need help opening snacks and some other two-handed tasks as well as help on the stairs. Emily had an easy time ascending and descending stairs—so long as she had a railing to hold on to. The problem was that handrails are typically only on one side of a stairwell. So if it was on her left side going up, she was fine, but she would need help coming down as it would then be on her right side. Dave went to Home Depot one day when Emily was three years old to get a handrail to install on our wall next to the stairs so that Emily always had a rail to hold on to. He came back with PVC piping and metal fittings. "What in the world?" I wanted to know what plumbing project he was working on.

"The handrails seemed so big for Emily's little hand," he explained. "She can grip this rubber PVC pipe much easier." So we had PVC pipes coming out of our walls on our staircase, but Emily could freely go up and down our stairs without needing our help.

Parenting Emily when she was healthy felt like, we guessed, parenting any child. She went to several doctor appointments a week and handled them with ease. If we had to wait, she drew pictures in her notebook and had no problem telling the doctor, "You're late." Beyond this, Emily was a typical little girl. She was smart—knew every letter of the alphabet and what sound it made when she was just three years old. Emily was never interested in growing her hair long, instead keeping it in the chin-length bob she had since her hair grew back from the chemotherapy. She could untangle a necklace and place it over her head with one hand before you could say, *Do you need help with that?* And she was girly! Her favorite things to play with were dolls and her play kitchen. But she countered the girly stuff with her love of baseball. She could throw more accurately at age three than most kids can at age 10. She also appreciated the satisfaction of hitting a plastic baseball to the other side of the yard—swinging that plastic bat with just one arm. Dave and I would often joke about her freakishly strong left arm.

Emily was now healthy and thriving and living a happy life. This meant that I was happy and living an easier life too. But I couldn't shake the undercurrent of stress from wondering if the tumor was going to grow back. It was always there, in the back and sometimes the front of my mind. And every three months I would find out on the eagerly anticipated MRI day and then breathe easier for a few more days. Then the stress crept back and I would have to wait another three months to breathe easier for a few days. As my sister-in-law once commented, it would be so much easier if there were a little window in her head.

We did have her physical limitations to manage daily. We still needed to fully dress her, open all her snacks, and help her with any other two-handed tasks. Helping her with these things was all we knew; it wasn't until we were around typically developing kids that we were more aware of Emily's differences. When Emily wanted to climb the jungle gym, I had to go with her—holding her hand as she navigated the stairs or rock wall to the top. So it was me and all the preschoolers hanging out on the playground equipment while the other moms sat on the park benches chit-chatting with each other. Or watching another child open her baggie of Goldfish and walk around eating them ... while I had to open Emily's bag then have her sit down and put the bag on her lap so that she could eat them. Those moments, the reminders of being different, felt isolating. It also made me wonder, if I was feeling like this just as Emily's "helper," what was Emily feeling like?

When Emily's good friend invited her to her gymnastics-themed birthday party at a trampoline gym, I broke down. Emily couldn't do gymnastics or use trampolines. I stressed over this party for days and even contemplated declining the invitation. But this was one of Emily's best friends and her mom was my close friend. I worried that Emily would feel left out and that I would have to spend the party on a trampoline holding Emily's hand, surrounded by 10 four-year-olds, while all the other moms sat at a nearby table watching. We went to the party, though, knowing that this was going to be the first of many situations that I, and she, would have to deal with. Thankfully, it turned out that the staff at the gym did everything they could to accommodate Emily's needs, and Emily seemed to not be fazed by any of her differences. I never once had to stand on the trampoline with her and I got to sit with the other moms and cheer as Emily bounced and rocked her floor routine—a series of endless twirls.

Emily seemed to have a great attitude about her differences. She was aware she only used one hand and other kids used two hands. She knew that she had a little more trouble with balance than the others. She couldn't ride a bike or a scooter like her friends liked to do. And although no one would ever think she was bothered by this, myself included, there were a handful of times that she admitted that her life was hard. As I tucked her in one particular night, Emily looked forlorn and whispered, "I wish my other hand worked. I don't like that I'm different."

Taken aback, all I could think to say was "I'm sorry, Em. It's not fair, is it?"

"No."

"But you can do so many things with just one hand! Not many people could do what you can do with just one hand. And you can run and jump and play like all of your friends."

Emily started crying. Inside, it felt like my heart was breaking into pieces. I held back my own tears and let her cry, holding her tight. She, of all people, had every right to cry. I flailed with how to help her.

After a few minutes I finally told her, "You can cry for a few more minutes if you want to. After that, you need to dry your eyes and think of all the happy things in your life."

She immediately wiped her tears away and listed her friends she liked to play with, her cat, and all her dolls. I added items to her list, like her grandparents, aunts, uncles and cousins who loved playing with her. I added what a great cook she was and how fast she could run. I told her how smart and funny she was. She was yawning now, and I was emotionally drained. That was the first time, and wouldn't be the last time, she admitted that being different took a toll on her. Those were the moments that were hardest for me to bear. I learned I could endure a lot, but watching my child suffer emotionally was hardest.

⇒ 8 ⇐

Grown Up Friends

We got the dreaded news during one of Emily's routine MRI appointments—the tumor was growing. She was now in her second year of preschool, and again, doing so well. We had noticed that when Emily was relaxing, her head tilted to the side, and she would choke a bit on her water after drinking. And even though it rattled in the back of our brains that perhaps those things were related to the tumor, I found it easy to brush aside. We could address these symptoms, if in fact they were symptoms, at the next doctor visit. She wasn't in pain and her life was not affected otherwise. The power of denial, of just wanting to continue our regular, normal life, was so strong that I was actually shocked to hear the news. I just nodded as the oncologist showed me the films and the measurements proving that the tumor had indeed grown. I sat there listening, the disbelief and surprise whittled away second by second, as he suggested radiation this time to treat the tumor. The technology had finally advanced and the new machine had just been installed at the main hospital. They could now more easily pinpoint the radiation and reduce the risk of damaging healthy tissue. He'd make an appointment for Dave and me to meet with the radiology team to discuss next steps. "Okay," I replied in my matter-of-fact tone. Still no emotion—Emily was with me and I didn't want to cue her that she should be sad about anything or have her be upset over me being sad. But I couldn't help the tears minutes later as I was navigating out of the parking garage, wondering the fate of Emily's future. "What's wrong, Mommy?" I heard a sweet, high voice ask.

"Oh, I just hurt my finger, but I'm fine," I quickly replied and wiped away my tears, gaining fake composure for the rest of the ride home.

Once I got home and busied Emily, I broke the news to Dave. He seemed to immediately go into denial that the tumor had grown by just brushing off my announcement and carrying on with what he was working on. I ended the conversation by saying, "I'm just telling you what the doctor said. We'll be meeting with the radiologist soon." I didn't press it because denial was a great place to be rather than our reality. I wished I could have still been there with him.

We met with the radiation oncologist a few days later. This doctor explained that they would use a beam of radiation directed exactly at the tumor to treat the cancer. He went on to explain that radiation would start working as soon as treatment was given as well as continue to work ... even years from now. The good news was that there would really be no side effects other than fatigue and dry skin/hair at the radiation site. The bad news was that she would need this treatment every day, Monday through Friday, for six straight weeks, and she would need anesthesia for each treatment as she would need to lie incredibly still as it was imperative there was no movement. Both Dave and I listened to the doctor talk, numbly nodding, with barely any emotion. We would start the following Monday.

I went to work the next day and explained the situation to my supervisor. I wanted to know if I could take six weeks of unpaid leave, starting Monday. This was *exactly* the kind of situation I dreaded when it came to my job. I hated asking for time off, especially since it wasn't a choice—I was going to take it whether they granted it to me or not—and now I had to ask for six weeks off. I was up most of the night before, not so much worrying about Emily's health, but nervous to have this conversation with my boss.

"No," was the response I received. Without missing a beat, my supervisor said, "You will take paid leave and use the sick leave pool." The leave pool was something that the employees all "paid" into each year by donating a vacation day to be used when situations like this arose for a colleague or themselves, like in my case. The good fortune I felt at that moment was a feeling I would never forget. I couldn't wait to get home and tell Dave. We had already begun trying to figure out what to cut out or scrimp on without my salary coming in or, worst-case scenario, I lost my job. With my salary still coming in and my job secure, all we had to worry about now was our four-year-old daughter receiving six weeks of radiation treatment to her brain.

The next day I went back to the hospital with Emily and my neighbor, Vicki, for the pre-radiation meeting. It was during this meeting that they molded a mask to fit on Emily's head that she would wear during the treatment. The mask, with Emily inside of it, would literally be clamped to the table to ensure no movement while they radiate an exact location each time. I never actually saw the mask, just the mold of Emily's face and head. Vicki, though, saw the mask at the end of the appointment (my back was to the room where they were creating it). When I asked her what it looked like since I was having a hard time picturing it, she said, "You don't want to know. Just don't look at it." She had a tone to her voice that meant she was not kidding, and I never saw the mask until they gave it to us as a keepsake at the end of her treatment. Vicki was right; there was no need for me to picture Emily with this mask on, strapped to a table. It looked like a Jason mask from the *Friday the 13th* horror movie series.

On Monday, Emily and I were out the door at 6 a.m. to get to the hospital and checked in by 7 for her first radiation treatment. Never had we been greeted with such enthusiasm and kindness than that morning at the radiation clinic. The staff who checked us in acted like we were long lost family members they were welcoming into their home for the first time, giving us a grand tour of the waiting rooms and restrooms. Wow, I thought, they really put out the red carpet for children, or maybe they just noticed that I was completely anxiety ridden and tried to calm my nerves. Either way, Emily felt like a queen and I relaxed. When it was Emily's turn, we walked into the back area where nurses accessed her mediport to give the anesthesia. Once the medicine was administered and she was asleep, I went back to the waiting room. In that room I could have a cup of coffee, watch *Dawson's Creek* playing on the TV, do a puzzle that was scattered on a table or read the variety of books that were placed throughout the room. I chose to just sit with my cup of coffee and people watch, trying to imagine everyone else's story. An hour later, I was called back to sit with Emily as she woke up from the anesthesia. Once she was fully awake, we were able to go home.

That afternoon, we stayed home, and I watched her like a hawk to see if there were any residual effects from the treatment that morning. But she had lunch, played with toys, watched some

TV, then helped me make dinner. She was herself—not even that tired.

The next morning, again at the hospital at 7, we were greeted with the exact same level of enthusiasm by the staff of the clinic. The exact same routine occurred, minus the tour of the waiting room, and we were home by 11 a.m. That afternoon, I took Emily to her preschool class since she was feeling good and wanting to go. This became our routine for six solid weeks. On the road at 6 a.m. to radiation for 7, home at 11 a.m., preschool at 1 p.m. and back home by 3:30. Emily felt fine during the entire treatment program. In fact, most people at school had no idea she was going through radiation treatment in the mornings.

We had to wait several more weeks for an MRI to see how the tumor looked after radiation. The results were good—the tumor hadn't grown and in fact had gone down in size slightly. As happy as I was to have this chapter behind us, the whole radiation therapy process seemed easy on Emily—and on me. Compared to brain surgery and chemotherapy, it was a breeze.

After Emily's radiation treatment was finished, I found myself in a good groove at work. I made strides with the projects I was assigned and worked with more and more people in the division, although they didn't know much about my personal life. I wanted to prove to everyone else that I was a professional. I was sensitive about having a different schedule than my co-workers—working from home a few days a week was not a common practice. And I didn't want people pitying me. I wanted to be treated equally, except for my schedule—I needed the flexibility and, honestly, I didn't mind being pitied to get that. But I didn't care if everyone else worked from home too! Mostly, though, I felt that people talked to or looked at me differently once they learned I had a child with cancer going through treatment. Suddenly, they didn't talk to me about their kids' accomplishments or struggles. Suddenly, I wasn't approachable. Suddenly, I was one of those moms that other moms gave the *that's got to be tough* nod and smile and then went on with their day without me because I was seemingly so different from them. I was lonely at work because of this. I missed the university and all the people who knew me "Before Diagnosis."

After a few months of settling into my role and keeping my

personal life close to the cuff, I eventually did start to get to know some of my colleagues, but not many. Most had a general understanding of Emily's medical condition because I was absent for six weeks during Emily's radiation. One of my kind colleagues who did learn of Emily's diagnosis arranged for Emily to be granted a trip to Disney World through a foundation she regularly volunteered with (the foundation granted trips to children who had significant medical challenges). When she first told me about it, suggesting it for Emily, I politely declined. I knew what a trip like that would cost and didn't feel comfortable accepting such a large gift. But she persisted and the next thing I knew I received a letter in the mail giving me the dates of our vacation.

Before we went, though, we were to attend a fundraising event where Emily was the star and it was here where we would officially receive the gift. I felt like I should have been jumping up and down screaming like a game show contestant who just won the grand prize. But I never signed up for this game show. I never wanted Emily to

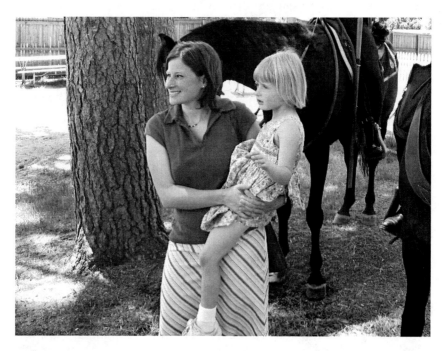

Emily and I having just received our gift of a trip to Disney World. Photograph by Jeff Daniels.

be in this situation. I didn't like being in the spotlight. I didn't want special treatment and certainly not pity. Dave felt like I did, only, it seemed, ten times worse. Don't get me wrong, we were grateful. We knew Emily would love the trip and we knew we couldn't afford it otherwise. But it was so hard to fight against our instincts to not draw attention to ourselves; we just wanted to be *normal*. Dave didn't even ask for the day off to attend the event and instead went to work. I didn't argue with him because I totally understood. I went with my family who was cheering us on while I plastered on a fake smile. Emily, however, welcomed the spotlight, which was always a comfortable place for her.

In the end we did go on that trip and truly appreciated all the people who donated time and money to make these sorts of trips happen. It turned out to be an incredible experience that gave us memories Emily talked about often. Her favorite story, by far, comes from the first day of this vacation. We came across the Tower of Terror ride which had no line, was inside, and had no height or age requirements. I was not familiar with the ride, but, other than the name, it sounded perfect—I was hot and tired, ready to sit down in some air conditioning. We climbed into this ride, set up to look like an elevator, and sat in one of the dozen seats available facing the elevator doors. We got Emily buckled into the seat between Dave and me and the ride started. This "elevator" dropped several floors with the door open and I lost my mind. It then shot up and dropped again at which point I screamed like a banshee. And then I started crying, feeling like the worst mother *ever* by bringing my sweet four-year-old on this horrific ride. I tried putting myself on top of Emily's lap to protect her and assure her this was all make-believe. Instead, as I laid on her lap, still shaking, bawling, and screaming, she was the one who patted my head and said, "It's okay, Mommy" and "It's almost over, Mommy" repeatedly until the ride ended. I was clearly reminded who the brave one in the family was, and she never let me forget it. We now view moments of generosity like this trip, which provided lasting memories, as one of the silver linings of Emily's diagnosis.

Shortly after that trip, during a particularly long day of sitting at my desk with not much work to do and no one to talk with, I walked to the stairwell. I worked on the fourth floor in a windowless space and started walking down to the lobby and back up to the fourth floor for a little exercise and a change of scenery whenever I needed a break. This time, though, I came across a colleague I was just starting to get to know sitting on the stairs looking just as miserable as I felt. I asked if she was okay and she smiled and shrugged. So I sat with her and we started sharing war stories from our jobs, complaining about certain colleagues and work dynamics. Typical work drama. Pretty soon we were laughing at ourselves and our pathetic routine of walking the stairwell to get away from our desks. She invited me out for drinks with her and her girlfriends that weekend.

I was excited to get out and spent way too long trying to figure out what to wear. Elisa was a few years younger than me, lived in the city, and wasn't married and didn't have kids. Her friends were probably the same. Adding to my stress of not knowing what to wear was that we were meeting at a bar in Denver (downtown!). Most of my socializing up to this point had been in my kitchen, in my neighbor's kitchen, or at the hospital. This was going to be the real deal. I had just gotten my hair cut and thought I looked like a 1950s housewife, which added to my anxiety of coming across to these new people like the suburban mom I was. But I got there and met my new friend Elisa, who introduced me to all her friends—a few I even knew from work—and they complimented my hair. They were probably just being polite, but it worked. I was at ease. I had a fun night meeting new people, who were definitely *not* suburban and all cooler than me, as well as getting to know Elisa better.

My friendship with Elisa continued to grow as we would have lunch together at work and a few more "girls' nights" she invited me to. I invited her to my house to hang out with us some weekends and we got into a routine of sitting on my deck with a drink, sometimes Dave joining us, sometimes not. She would always play with Emily and had a great rapport with her. Elisa was laid-back and easy to be with, sometimes easier to be with than other "mom" friends since I didn't have to worry about kids getting along, bringing Emily to another house where I had to be "on duty" and not able to relax in case there were stairs she needed to go up or down, toys she needed two hands to play with, etc. But mostly, we could talk about real life and I could be myself, my normal self. I let her know the details of Emily's life. She listened, asked questions, and was helpful, but she didn't pity me. She talked to me about her life, let me listen and ask questions and try to be helpful when I could. And we could laugh. We laughed *a lot*.

Early in our friendship I had a particularly bad day—I had left work early to bring Emily to an unexpected doctor appointment, got pulled over for speeding, and once back home proceeded to spill my travel mug of coffee down my shirt. Elisa had just come over as I ran upstairs to change my shirt. When I returned, Elisa was completing her lesson on how to make Mommy a gin and tonic. Emily proudly announced, "I squeezed the lime!" I shook my head and laughed at Elisa for thinking that was appropriate. She exclaimed it was a great life lesson that was essential in my household. She was not wrong.

As my friendship with Elisa blossomed, so did friendships with a few others from work. We would get together for girls' nights out every so often as well as have lunch together at work. I would let them into my world, and they let me into their worlds. There was no judgment or pity once I let these people in, I soon realized, just real friendship.

One afternoon, while catching up with Elisa at her desk, Elisa asked me how a doctor appointment for Emily went. Elisa's office-mate interrupted, wanting clarification as to what I was talking about. And after I gave her a condensed version of Emily's diagnosis and treatment, all with a comforting smile on my face—which I had learned to do when people asked me these things—she blurted out, "But you're so normal!"

I didn't know how to respond. Was that a compliment? *Of course I'm normal!* is what I wanted to shout with annoyance. Was I not supposed to be able to have a job or have friends or laugh? It was at that point I no longer doubted that I was viewed differently by some people; I knew it. I understood, though. I, too, had viewed other parents of special needs children before I had Emily as people I couldn't relate to, and, therefore, different. In the end, I responded to Elisa's officemate with a simple "I guess so."

Later, as Elisa apologized to me for her officemate's comment, I learned that people at work who didn't know me, just knew that I had a daughter with a brain tumor, referred to me as the "Ice Queen." They knew about Emily's diagnosis, but since I didn't talk about it much or appear upset when they saw me, they concluded that I had ice running through my veins. I knew I should have been offended by the name. I wasn't, though. I had been through too much to let simple name calling get to me. (I wish I had been this strong in middle school.) The only thing it did was make me second guess how to act. Do I openly talk about my home life or not? I never figured out the right answer.

Emily was finishing up her last year of preschool and feeling great. The MRIs were looking good since her radiation treatment. Dave and I were comfortable in our jobs and our relationship. We were surrounded by friends. My parents had even moved to Colorado and lived just 10 minutes away. Dare I say, life was looking up. We had several months to believe this—time enough to start looking forward, not just live in the now.

Both Dave and I grew up with siblings and imagined that for Emily as well. Not just for childhood years, but for adulthood. My brothers are about a decade older than me. They like to say I was the "oops" baby; I like to say I was the "pleasant surprise." Needless to say, due to that age difference, we didn't play together like typical siblings when I was growing up. In fact, I was too young to even remember when all three of us all lived together at home. But the boys always came home for weekend visits or my parents and I would spend a week with my brothers wherever they may have been living. And Mike married Kim when I was just 11 years old. So, in all respects, Kim is not just a sister-in-law but a sister to me.

Despite the miles that were always between us, we talked with each other regularly. Dave jokingly states that we have a "Daniels Hotline" that gets activated for any type of news (whether it be Jeff made it safely to Tibet or Dad decided to plant a rose garden). And since I had Emily, experiencing Mike, Kim and Jeff rally around me and Dave proved how important it was for Emily to have a sibling.

Dave, on the other hand, grew up with three siblings all within a year or so of each other. They were his playmates day in and day out. He even shared a room with his brother during his entire childhood. And although Dave drifted away from his family (the only one to move out of state), he had fond memories of playing with his sisters and brother growing up.

We also didn't think we were done parenting. It was a silly thought when our child was only five years old, but with Emily starting school full-time soon, we felt like a big chapter was closing that we did not want to close. But we worried. Would we have another child with medical issues? Unfortunately, we were now acutely aware of how many things could go wrong. We were also too informed of what that life was like—for both the child and the parent. Did we want to take that risk? And, of course, the timing was never great. When Dave would bring up the idea of having another baby, I was quick to dismiss it—either Emily was still undergoing treatment or just recovering from a surgery of some sort. Then, when I would bring up the idea, he would squash it for the very same reasons. That summer before Emily started kindergarten, though, we were both in sync on the idea of having another baby. Both of us felt very optimistic about Emily's future, and the brain tumor was not a part of it.

Within moments, it seemed, of making the decision to have a baby, I found out I was pregnant. It must have been kismet and we were overjoyed. Well, cautiously overjoyed. I played the odds—what were the chances this baby could have a significant medical issue? My gut told me slim to none and I easily felt that this baby was going to be healthy. Dave, though, was going through this pregnancy with me from a step away, shielding his heart. Happy, excited, doing all the dad things, yes, but with a bit more reserved nature, not wanting to get too attached.

We shared the news with everyone early, at around 10 weeks. This was mostly because I was tired and already starting to show. And frankly, people were a bit suspicious of me turning down drinks for two months straight. My parents were shocked we felt brave enough to try this again but were thrilled at the idea of it. As usual, they would support anything we wanted to do. We told Emily that we were going to have a baby and she announced that she would like a sister. Not surprising for the little girl who always had a doll close by that she dressed in pink, frilly clothes on a regular basis.

My prenatal appointments were, thankfully, uneventful. The only hard part of this pregnancy was reducing the fierce caffeine habit I now had. I went from drinking five to six cups of coffee a day to one cup a day and that was torturous.

Emily started kindergarten at the end of the summer. She was going to a full day program at our neighborhood public school (the same place she went for preschool) and I don't know which of us was more excited. This smart, talkative, social, precocious little girl was going to be so happy to be around kids all day learning new things. And I was going to be without a kid for most of the day! I could now do things like work a full day and go to the grocery store without my little helper. I was not one of the moms who stood on the field waving goodbye to their five-year-old behind big sunglasses trying to hide the fact that they were crying. Nope, I was the one cheerfully waving goodbye with a big smile on my face. Emily was confident and ready to be around other people—as was I.

I had a quick meeting with the kindergarten teacher prior to her starting to explain that she only had use of one hand and would need help with two-handed tasks. I barely brought up the fact that Emily had a brain tumor. In my mind, that was a thing of the past. Her kindergarten teacher had taught for many years and was everything you want a kindergarten teacher to be—kind, understanding, and no nonsense. I confidently left Emily in her hands and I went to work, able to fully concentrate on my projects. At the end of that first day, though, I was anxiously waiting for Emily outside the school door. It turned out to be a long day and I was dying to know how her day went. The bell finally rang and Em marched out, promptly announcing while pointing at the door behind her, "There are *a lot* of rules in there!" But she concluded she would go back because she had fun too.

At 20 weeks into my pregnancy we got the ultrasound that showed us that the baby was healthy and a boy! I was thrilled and cracked up when I looked at Dave who said, "Oh no!" He remembered all the boy antics he pulled as a child and was terrified. "We've got this, it'll be great," I said. Here we were on another new adventure. We broke the news to Emily that night at dinner that she was going to have a little brother, not a sister. Thankfully, she was just as excited with this news as we thought she would be with a sister. She was thrilled to be on this new adventure as well.

The same week as my 20-week ultrasound, I had plans to meet up with some of my colleagues from the university. My former supervisor was in town and I was excited to get together with her and the old gang. I went to kiss Emily goodbye as she sat on Dave's lap and she proceeded to jerk her head to the side, lift her arm up to the sky, and kick her leg out. After about 30 seconds, she did this again, and then again a minute later. She was talking the whole time and seemed confused when I asked her what she was doing. I immediately looked at Dave and said, "I think she's having a seizure." To this day, I'm not sure where that thought came from as I had no experience or knowledge of seizures at that time.

"No, I don't think that's how seizures look." Dave responded. He reassured me that she was fine and encouraged me to leave so I wouldn't be late for my dinner. I hesitantly left and later, when I was with friends, I felt silly for thinking she had a seizure.

When I got home, Dave said she fell asleep shortly after I left at 5:30 p.m. We agreed that it was a bit of an odd behavior coming from her and I called the neuro-oncologist the next morning to tell him about it. He agreed with my initial assumption. "It probably was a seizure," he said. "Bring her in for a CT scan today. Let's make sure it wasn't prompted by a change in the tumor."

I couldn't believe he thought she had a seizure, not because I wanted to be right, but because she was supposed to be healthy now. This was not part of our new adventure plans. Neither was the possibility that the tumor was growing again. Thankfully, the CT scan showed that the tumor had not changed in size. We didn't know what had caused the seizure, but we needed to keep an eye on her to see if she would have any more.

Shortly after this one seizure occurred, the kindergarten teacher called to say Emily seemed very tired. She wondered if she was having sleepless nights. "No," I answered, "Emily seems to be sleeping all night long." The teacher pulled me aside the next day after school. "I think you should look into whether or not Emily is having seizures in the middle of the night, therefore disrupting her sleep. I had another student, years ago, who was very tired during the day and it was due to seizure activity during the night." I tucked her suggestion away. I trusted her input, but I so desperately wanted this seizure nonsense to end. I justified Emily's sleepiness during the day with her being in school for a full day rather than the two and a half hours of preschool she was used to. I was pregnant and wanted smooth sailing ahead— no more medical disruptions, please.

That same day at dinnertime Emily had another seizure like the first one we saw. I called the doctor back and told him about the new seizure and explained the sleepiness during the day. He then referred us to a pediatric neurologist. By the time we saw the neurologist she had about four seizures that we knew of. They all looked like her first one, except they lasted longer—closer to 10 minutes—and she immediately went to sleep afterwards.

The neurologist explained that she was having simple partial seizures, a type of seizure that Emily remained conscious through. He believed the kindergarten teacher was right; she probably was having them at night, interrupting her sleep. Although seizures make a person sleepy afterward, if you were sleeping when one started, it would fully wake you up. He also could not explain exactly why she was suddenly having them, but he stressed that we needed to treat her with medication to stop the seizures from occurring. Seizures themselves are not necessarily dangerous, but the accidents that could occur due to them can cause serious injury. For instance, Emily could be standing on an escalator at the mall, have a seizure, and fall. Seizures that last too long are also considered a medical emergency.

My easy pregnancy and lovely routine of Emily being in school all day, every day disappeared. I was using my sick and vacation days as fast as I earned them for the onslaught of Emily's new doctor appointments. And we were struggling with Emily's new reality of living with seizures. There really was no predicting when one would occur, abruptly stopping whatever it was she was doing and then bringing on a nap. I couldn't think, or believe, that this was going to be her (and our) future. We went back to thinking of only today and tomorrow.

In the midst of Emily's new diagnosis of epilepsy, she had a series of urinary tract infections (UTIs). She had started seeing a pediatric urologist who suggested she have tests done to see specifically what was causing the UTIs and therefore develop a successful treatment plan. One of the tests involved inserting a catheter for her to void through while a series of X-rays took images of the bladder. When they explained the X-ray part, I thought it meant one quick X-ray that I could easily step away from because I was pregnant. What I didn't quite understand was that they took a series of X-rays over several minutes, inserted a catheter, and then took another series of X-rays. It was an awful, painful test. Especially painful when you don't have your mommy next to you to say it's all right. I had to stand behind the glass and watch her cry during the test with my heart in my throat. After the test she just wiped her tears away and told the nurses, "I did not like that! Don't do that to me again!" My strong fighter—you tell 'em.

The test results confirmed that her right kidney refluxed causing bacterial infections. It was a condition most likely caused by her weakened right side, but easily treatable with a daily low-dose antibiotic. We just had to make sure it didn't progress or get worse.

As if this wasn't enough, she stopped growing. The tumor's location or the treatment for the tumor, difficult to tease out at this point, caused her to go into early puberty. We quickly got her on monthly injections at the doctor's office to stop puberty from progressing, and every night, in addition to giving her the pills in her pill box, I would give her an injection in her thigh of a growth hormone so that she would continue to grow.

Even through all of Emily's medical issues, she made it to her kindergarten class just about every day, even if it was just a half day. She continued to learn to read, make friends, and have play dates. And although she spent too much of her time at the hospital for various appointments and had a slew of diagnoses on her medical chart, she laughed and joked and was a genuine joy to be around (unless you were a medical professional which she had an uncanny ability to both charm and tell off).

Emily didn't complain about going to the doctor's office. She didn't feel sorry for herself. Her attitude absolutely made my job, as her mom, easier. I relied on her cues—her strong, happy spirit—to guide my attitude. I didn't break down because Emily didn't break down. Dave and I continued to work every day we could, even if just a few hours. We didn't see friends much as our energy levels were lower than ever, it seemed. But my pregnancy remained easy and we had this baby boy to look forward to. Assuming Emily's medical crises would stop.

⇒ 9 ⇐

Baby Time

A few months after Emily turned six years old, in the spring of her kindergarten year, Ryan was born. Everything went as planned, as planned as any birth could be anyway, and he was declared healthy. That same day, my parents brought Emily to visit us in the hospital and she beamed at the sight of her little brother. As soon as she approached him, she placed her hand on his bald head, then turned to my mom and whispered, "I hope his brain is okay." With tears in her eyes after hearing the apprehension in Emily's voice, none of us realizing Emily had this concern, my mom helped get her into my bed. Emily held Ryan in her arms and went into mama mode just as quickly as I did.

My first month home with Ryan was so much more relaxing than it was with Emily. We had sleepless nights, but not endless screaming. This baby just wanted his bottle and this baby drank the bottle. I knew right away and had no doubts that Ryan was healthy. It took Dave some time to truly believe it and was still a bit guarded initially. It took months for him to accept that Ryan was a relaxed baby who had a soft cry that typically stopped when you fed him.

When Ryan was just weeks old, I left him for four days while I took Emily to the hospital for an EEG study to track her seizure activity. I had to stifle my aching feelings to do this but couldn't imagine not being there for Emily as she had wires strung up to her head and was confined to her bed for four days. This was the first of many times I struggled with not being able to be with both of my babies—one of my worst struggles. Helping, though, was that Ryan was happy, healthy, and still sleeping a lot of the time—his four-week

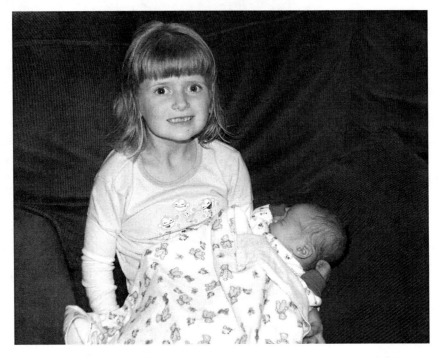

Emily, age six, holding her newborn baby brother, Ryan.

self still growing and growing. Emily was now six years old, having multiple seizures a week, the medicines not working.

Other than the heartache of leaving Ryan at home with Dave, the hardest part of the EEG study was entertaining an otherwise healthy six-year-old confined to a bed for four days straight. There are only so many board games to play, books to read, and pictures to draw before you want to jump out the window. Somehow, with the help of visitors, we got through that hospital stay. Emily cooperated by having seizures throughout our four days at the hospital, therefore making it not a waste of time—which was my other worry.

The results of the study resulted in a new regiment of medicines to try to control the seizures. They all needed time to work and then the dosage could be tweaked for more control. It was a very fluid and slow process that felt more like trial and error than actual science. Emily would try a new medicine and we would wait a few weeks to see if the seizures disappeared. When they didn't, we'd call the doctor back and he would prescribe a new medicine or dose and we'd wait a few more weeks to see if the seizures stopped.

This was about the same time I was supposed to go back to work, as my maternity leave was ending. And I couldn't fathom the thought of it. I had been working 32 hours a week, two days in the office and the rest of time at home, prior to my leave and I was supposed to return to that schedule next week. But Emily still had weekly physical and occupational therapy visits along with a barrage of new specialist appointments coming up. Plus, the biggest reason I couldn't imagine going back to work was I had a beautiful baby boy to take care of in between all those appointments. There were just not enough minutes in the day to attend to everything.

I started to panic thinking I couldn't juggle all the appointments and time with Ryan with work. I told Dave all my concerns, after a night of not sleeping, and he suggested that I call work and let them know I needed more time before I came back. "But what if I get fired? They have every right to lay me off since my maternity leave contract is up, and it states that I would return in the same capacity as before my leave."

"Well, then, you get fired," was his response. Ha! We both knew we needed my income, but we would have to figure that out later. One panic attack at a time. Right now, I knew I couldn't go back to work.

That afternoon I made the phone call to my boss. I told her everything, ending with my declaration that I just couldn't make it into the office next week and I didn't know when I could. She then asked, "Do you think you could work if it was just 20 hours a week and all from home?" After a pause to digest what she said, I responded, *"YES!"* and thanked her profusely as I didn't think that would be an option. I then quickly got off the phone before she could change her mind. This job had come a long way from the 8 a.m. to 5 p.m. that everyone was expected to work.

Mercifully, Emily's wait to get Medicaid was now over and we no longer had to pay her doctor copays, which helped ease the pain of me losing hours at work. It was incredible to wrap our minds around the fact that we no longer had to shell out $20 or $50 every time we stepped foot in a doctor's office for Emily. And that was on top of the premiums we paid into monthly for the top-of-line insurance we bought. With every cry from Emily, with every doctor stating we had to come back for another appointment, we couldn't help but weigh the cost of that appointment. Is Emily sick enough to bring her in to the specialist? Do we have the $50 to cover it? What if he prescribes another medication? How much is that going to cost? Not having that internal battle anymore was one of the biggest reliefs we ever experienced. I would gladly fill out the mountain of paperwork we had to do each year as well as endure quarterly home visits from a social worker to maintain Medicaid for Emily.

I felt a lot of stress leave me between being able to work from home and not having the financial burden of Emily's doctor's appointments. Plus, I had this sweet chunk of a little boy to cuddle. Ryan had a very calm demeanor and went with the flow. He was my real-life teddy bear I even nicknamed "Bear." I was not alone with my infatuation with him. Emily *loved* taking care of him, always in mommy mode. I would let her hold him on her lap and give him a bottle while I cleaned the kitchen or made dinner. She was truly a great help and Ryan was (and still is) a patient little brother. He would hang out on her bed among all her dolls, *E.T.*–style, while she played house or school. My best memories of Ryan as a baby took place in Emily's pink and green room, the three of us dancing to the *Lilo and Stitch* CD, which was full of Elvis and Hawaiian luau songs. We did that day in and day out for weeks at a time, the summer between Emily's kindergarten and first grade year.

Ryan, in stark contrast to Emily, was reaching every milestone exactly when the books said a baby should. Emily, though, was suffering from more and more seizures and needed constant supervision. It got to the point where I couldn't even let her hold Ryan on her lap if I wasn't sitting right next to her. We were still trying a variety of anti-seizure cocktails to get the right kind and dosage. She seemed to go a week or two without any seizures, and then they would start again. We would then try a new dose or set of medicines and watch what happened.

But the seizures kept happening and were unpredictable. We now had to accompany her on the stairs after she had a seizure while standing on the top of the stairs and fell all the way down. Luckily, she just got some bruises, but it scared me and terrified Dave. After that incident, I made her wake me up when she got up for the day so I could walk her downstairs to where the family room was. And since the seizures started, she started getting up earlier and earlier. After

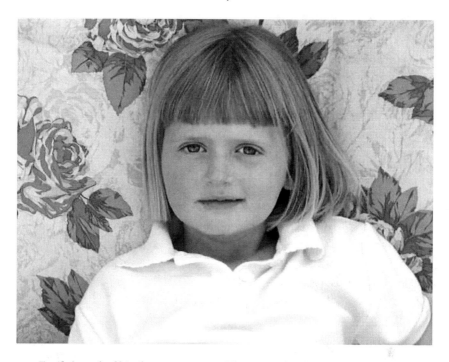

Emily's end of kindergarten year. Photograph taken by Jeff Daniels.

weeks of coming to get me in the middle of the night so she could go downstairs (and me telling her no and putting her back to bed every 15 minutes until I gave up), I finally told her that the first number on the clock had to say 5 (early, but better than 4 a.m.), 6 (this would be nice) or 7 (wishful thinking) before she could get out of bed. So at 5 on most mornings, she would wake me up, I would walk her down the stairs, sit her safely on the couch with instructions not to move, turn on the TV and go back to sleep until Ryan woke me up for the day—usually an hour later.

Fall was fast approaching, and I got a call from the school nurse to update her plan. Because of Emily's medical diagnosis and physical disability, she had an IEP (individualized education plan) in place. This is a plan that outlines what extra items Emily needs in school to be successful due to her specific circumstances. Up until now, things in her IEP stated things like the toilet paper roll holder needed to be on the left side of the stall; Emily may need additional time to use the restroom; Emily will have assistance during lunch to open her water bottle if needed; and so on. Those were protections for Emily that the school would accommodate. After I gave the nurse the update regarding Emily's still-uncontrolled seizure activity, the school suggested they add a need for a one-on-one aide to her IEP. This aide would assist her with all two-handed tasks as well as be there in case Emily had a seizure at school.

Getting Emily an aide sounded like a very reasonable, if not progressive, response from the school, but I wanted nothing to do with it and refused the aide. Emily was still as independent as most kids her age—just needed a little help here and there with two-handed tasks. If she had a seizure, she just needed to be seated to stay safe. That was it—in my mind she hardly needed accommodations. I was so used to accommodating her needs I stopped thinking of them being anything but ordinary. The school was adamant, though, that they hire an aide for her, at least for part of the day. I relented but relayed my worry that Emily would grow dependent on this person to do things for her instead of Emily trying for herself, losing her strong drive to be independent.

The school seemed to have listened. They hired a wonderful woman, a parent herself, who totally understood my concerns. This aide not only appreciated her spunk but helped make it thrive. With her aide's help, Emily got through her first-grade routine easily. She continued friendships with kids from her preschool days as well as made new friends. I noticed that Emily gravitated to the "wild child" of the group. These kids seemed to not give a damn what other people thought of them which translated into being secure enough to have friendships with someone who was outwardly different. Don't get me wrong, these were good kids—great kids, even. But these were kids who would question rules and not easily back down—and probably exhausted their parents day in and day out. And I loved them for loving my girl.

While Emily was in school, I easily got work done at home when Ryan played contently and during his naps, which he religiously took. If it was a hectic day or if a deadline was approaching, I worked in the evenings. Our experience with Ryan as a baby was so different than Emily, we decided we probably wouldn't have waited six years to have another baby if he had come first. He was low maintenance—happy with just some food and toys to play with.

But by the end of Emily's first grade year, we realized she was sleeping more than she was awake while in school. Every day she would have at least one seizure and proceed to nap on the bean bag chair the teacher had set up for her in the quiet reading corner. She had also begun to lose control of her bladder during seizures which was, of course, quite embarrassing for her. Amazingly, though, she mostly kept up with her schoolwork. She learned to read and do simple math. She put together a project on jungle animals that she presented to the class. At home, in between seizures, she played house, bossed around her baby brother, and worked hard to make him laugh.

We noticed, though, our daily routines started to revolve around epilepsy. It was proving to be an incredible hardship on Emily's life and, therefore, our lives. The not knowing when a seizure would occur, and then dealing with the aftermath of it, made planning anything very difficult. I didn't feel comfortable letting Emily go over to friends' houses for playdates anymore for fear she would have a seizure then need to sleep, effectively ending the playdate. Of course, this meant that her friendships were dwindling. A simple trip to the grocery store was no longer simple. She could have a seizure. And if she had one, we'd have to find a place for her to sit *and* get her there safely. At six years old, it was no longer easy to just pick her up and carry her. Dave and I both experienced a few exasperated trips out with her. With unsaid words, we started doing errands on our own— the other was left at home with Emily. We hated epilepsy.

It was at this time the neurologist suggested we think about surgery to resect the area of her brain that the seizures were originating from. She was having an average of four seizures a day and the anti-seizure medicines were obviously not working. The doctor had tried without success for more than a year now to find a mix that would work and this was the next line of treatment available.

The doctor was able to pinpoint the area of her brain that the seizures were coming from with the EEG tests Emily had undertaken over the last year. That area, in typical developing brains, was the area that speech comes from and this was what the doctor was most concerned about. He could do this surgery, but she could lose her speech. The good news was that Emily's brain was most likely wired differently. She was very high functioning which led the doctor to believe she was using different areas of the brain to compensate for the damage from the tumor. This was common with children who suffered brain injuries—they could, essentially, rewire their brain. The doctor relayed that he could find out what this area of the brain controlled by having her do a functional MRI.

We agreed to go forward with this specialized MRI. But there was a hurdle—there were only two MRI machines in the country that could take functional images. One was in Texas and the other in New York City. Although Texas was closer to us, the neurologist had done his residency at the hospital in New York, where one of the functional MRI machines was, and knew the doctors involved, so we chose to go to that one. Our insurance plan, however, had a different idea. They denied the functional MRI altogether, stating it wasn't necessary. Medicaid would not cover this out-of-state test either. I proceeded to spend more than three weeks on the phone with insurance agents pleading our case, even having doctors here and doctors in New York write urgent letters to the insurance company stating the need for this type of testing. Yet the insurance group was not budging.

I was hearing radio silence from the insurance group at this point and Emily's seizure activity was worsening. Dave and I were forced to finally talk about this disease that we had been living with but not talking about. It seemed to progress gradually enough that we just went through the motions of managing it. The countless doctor appointments, the number of times one of us said "she had a seizure" to explain her sleeping on the couch again, or the times one of us ran out to the grocery store after bedtime to avoid taking her seemed to just turn into routine. But we hated this routine. And we decided it was no life for Emily. We couldn't imagine her living like this much longer.

We went ahead and scheduled the MRI, prepared to pay the $1,000 for the test along with the incredibly pricey 24-hour trip to NYC (with a huge sigh of relief, we got word minutes before Emily had the scan that insurance would cover the test). Yet again, I was leaving my baby boy at home. It wasn't any easier. But between his mellow demeanor and Emily's seizure activity worsening, I tried not to dwell on it. Emily and I got through the long security line at Denver International Airport, stopped for a treat of McDonald's for breakfast, and then walked toward our gate. We had to sit, literally, in the middle of the floor of the hallway on our way to the gate while Emily had a seizure. I sat next to her, one hand on her back, one on our suitcase, the bag of McDonald's on my lap, and watched as strangers jogged by trying to catch their flight. I endured the looks we got—both of annoyance and curiosity—as we sat blocking the path of people for the 15 minutes of Emily's seizure. I knew the odds of this happening and left for the airport one hour earlier than I normally would have. I wasn't stressed. And, by now, I was hardened enough to not let the looks bother me.

I've always loved New York City—the lights, the activity, the buildings, the people watching—it was all endless. I was excited to be there even if it was for a doctor's appointment. After we settled into our room, we walked to the corner restaurant and had a slice of pizza like any tourist would do in the city. But then Emily had another seizure and was tired. Back to the room we went where Emily ended up just going to bed for the night. I pulled a chair up to the window and sat for the remainder of the night watching all the people go by, wondering what their lives were like. Did they live here? Or are they on vacation? Are they heading to a show tonight? I became wistful and sad, understanding that life with Emily meant I could not do the things the people outside the window were doing. I continued to sit, pondering the what ifs of life as the sky grew dark and the lights came on.

Dave and I by now had a very limited social life. We used to get together with our neighborhood friends at our house most weekends. It was easy for them to stop by and have a beer or share a meal—they had small kids too. But some were moving away, including my good friend Vicki, and we saw them less and less, really not much at all these days. Our friends Steve and Sonja added to their family as well, with a little girl Ryan's age, and we saw them on occasion—they lived half an hour away from us and it was sometimes hard to schedule a day when they weren't busy. Dave and I rarely made an effort to go out ourselves. We just weren't comfortable hiring a babysitter. Explaining Emily's situation without causing panic and fear was difficult. Instead, we relied on people who were close to us to watch the kids, like my parents, brothers, or Elisa. They all had lives, too, and were often busy on weekends themselves. I felt bad asking them to cancel their plans, so Dave and I sat at home by ourselves most of the time, sitting on our deck or watching TV. On those occasions when my parents did come over to babysit or Elisa offered, we were giddy with excitement. I would practically spring out of bed the morning of our night out and be in a great mood all day, looking forward to being a grown-up that night and leaving all my worries behind. But when the night came and we were out at a restaurant either by ourselves or with some friends, I realized that I just wasn't carefree anymore—there was no leaving my worries behind. I wasn't as quick to laugh as our friends and couldn't easily bound from bar to bar without looking at my watch, knowing I would need to be functioning by 5 a.m. the next day. It was hard for me to unwind, hard to shove the doctor's appointments, the diagnosis, and the knowledge of how difficult Emily's life was, aside in order to have a good time. I missed being able to fully enjoy a night out without the worry of Emily's health lingering in my head. So as I watched these people in New York City, walking about with the lights twinkling around them, I was enveloped in pure envy and longing.

The next morning, as I hailed a cab to take us to the hospital for the functional MRI, Emily had another seizure. I was busy holding on to her when the cab pulled in. I opened the door and said to the driver, "Hang on—it will take me a second to get her in the car."

"What's going on?" he asked.

"She's having a seizure, but it's all right. I can get her in in a second."

He shrugged in movie scene New York City fashion as I worked to get her in the cab. She slept the 30-minute drive to Columbia, and I breathed a sigh of relief that she had a seizure then. It most likely meant she wouldn't have one when we got to the hospital. I had never been to this hospital before and we probably had a lot of walking around to do before finding exactly where we needed to be. If she had a seizure, then it would just add to the chaos. Once we were dropped off at the entrance, I found the building we were supposed to go to, walked in and proceeded down the hallway, following the signs, to the doctors who would be working with us. In just a matter of minutes, Emily was in the MRI machine easily going through their battery of tests. Two hours later we were in a black car on our way back to the airport.

We resumed our regular routine once we got home while waiting for the results of the MRI. Emily went to school, Dave worked his three-day work week, I worked at home a few hours each day and hung out with Ryan the rest of the time. Ryan and I picked Emily up from our neighborhood school every day. And every day the teacher would tell me that Emily had a seizure (or two) and napped afterward. The teacher was very sympathetic and did a great job of letting Emily take a quiet moment when needed and inviting her back to the lesson when she felt ready. Emily never quite remembered the seizures or the aftermath but still reported on the remainder of her day and took part in plenty of the learning activities.

The kids in first grade split up for reading and math and Emily was in the other first grade teacher's class for reading. Right after our trip to New York for the functional MRI, Emily's reading teacher called me in for a conference. They had just completed their schoolwide testing and she was concerned about Emily's scores. She proceeded to show me the poor results of her standardized test and casually mentioned that she had a seizure prior to taking the test. Taken aback, I explained, "She should not have been tested at that time. She was probably extremely fatigued and disoriented if she just had a seizure."

That seemed to fall on deaf ears as the reading teacher proceeded to give me tips to help Emily score better on these types of tests. "Emily didn't recognize this picture of a baseball player. Do you take her to ball games? Maybe you should take her out more and let her explore the world a bit."

I reiterated that she had a seizure prior to the test. She continued with her lecture on how important it is to take children out into the world to explore new things. In my head, I told this teacher that Emily had probably been to more places in her seven years than she had her entire life all while battling a brain tumor and epilepsy. Instead, I nodded and said, "Sure, I'll just take her to a ball game, and she should surely score better on her reading test." She was pleased with my answer. I'm pretty sure she didn't detect my sarcasm. She was the least of my worries, though.

One week after Emily's functional MRI test in New York we received the results. She didn't use the area of the brain that her seizures were originating from for speech, reading, math, logic or any of the other testing that was done, which meant surgery was an option. It was, again, decision time for Dave and me. She had been through brain surgeries before and we knew what they entailed. The thought of her living with the number of seizures she was having made it clear that we needed to do something. She couldn't go on like this. We gave the go-ahead to do the surgery over the summer break.

As I did with any doctor appointment, I didn't make it a big deal in front of Emily. In fact, I didn't mention anything to her until the day before her surgery. I kept it light with just the bare minimum, telling her she would have a procedure to help stop the seizures and that we would stay in the hospital for a few days. That was it. That was all I wanted her seven-year-old mind to process and to think about. She balked this time about being in the hospital overnight. After the EEG "sleepover" she caught on that hospital stays were boring. But she was also turning into that model first child—wanting to please and not make waves. Her protests were small and short-lived. Twenty minutes later she was running through the front yard playing a game of tag with the neighborhood kids and in good spirits. Dave would always joke with Emily about her skinny legs, saying she had "chicken legs." As she was running around that night, I asked her what we should have for dinner and she quickly lifted her pant leg up and yelled, "chicken legs!"

≋ 10 ≋

Goodbye Epilepsy

The troops were rallied for yet another surgery. My whole family lived in Colorado by now and they all showed up for varying shifts during the long wait. Signing the consent forms was different this time and I was in denial that anything could go wrong. They were removing a piece of brain that was not being used for anything. That's what went through my head—that and how amazing it would be to not have to worry about seizures anymore. How Emily didn't have to face a future of epilepsy medications and constant worry of having a seizure. How I would be able to drop her off at a friend's house and not say she might have a seizure, this is what they look like, this is what you do if she has one. And I wouldn't have to see the look of panic across the other mom's face as I was explaining her condition. I thought how much Emily would excel at school if she could be awake for class. I also selfishly thought how much easier my life would be not having to deal with seizures. I thought how great it would be to go out somewhere with both Ryan and Emily and not having to plop Ryan on the ground, hoping he wouldn't crawl away, so I could hold onto Emily while she had a seizure. But most of all, I wanted Emily to have an easier life.

Emily got through this surgery with flying colors. Her recovery in the ICU was limited to just one night. And, best of all, the ICU unit had been improved. There were private (window-walled) rooms with a reclining chair for the parent. Plus, you were now allowed to sleep next to your child in the ICU. Such a seemingly small thing, but it meant the world to me that I wouldn't have to leave my child's side at her sickest times.

As soon as the breathing tube came out that night in the ICU, she asked for juice. We high-fived everyone we could reach. Her speech was not affected! I thought the worst was over. I was wrong.

She went straight to a private room on the fifth floor for the remainder of her stay. On the second night, she had a seizure. I deflated a bit, but not much. Perhaps this was just due to the trauma of the surgery. The neurologist agreed to let her heal completely before calling this procedure a failure. I was still optimistic and looking forward to a seizure-free future. Denial was a wonderful friend.

The rest of the hospital stay was uneventful. She was older now and enjoyed the attention from the nurses and everyone else who visited, especially the therapy dogs. I was even able to get a major report for work done and emailed to my colleague to submit. We had the usual sets of visitors throughout the week, including Mike and Kim. This time, though, they brought me a chilled tumbler. Confused, used to getting delivered a cup of coffee, I asked, "What's this?"

Kim replied, "I thought you would enjoy this instead of coffee. Take a sip!"

I hesitantly took a drink and then grinned like a Cheshire cat. It was a gin and tonic. My favorite summertime drink.

A few days later, Emily and I were discharged. After my big reunion with Ryan, I bathed Emily and had her lie down on the couch in the family room while I cooked dinner. She asked, "What's for dinner?"

"Mac and cheese," I responded.

Not one minute later, she asked, "What's for dinner?"

I said "Mac and cheese" a little louder this time because she clearly didn't hear me.

Two minutes went by and Emily asked, "What's for dinner?"

I laughed this time and said, "You're funny."

She ignored me and asked again, "What's for dinner?"

Dave, who was sitting in the family room with her, said, "I don't think she remembers. I think her memory is gone." I looked at him in disbelief. And then I thought about all the repeated conversations we had in the hospital. All the times she asked how long she would have to stay in the hospital. Maybe it *wasn't* just because she was anxious to go home; maybe she just couldn't remember the answer.

I didn't know what to think of this development. Was this

temporary? What would this mean? It had to be temporary. She had major surgery six days ago and still needed to heal.

The next day was filled with a lot of repetitive questions but she seemed a bit better. And each day did feel a little better. However, she definitely had trouble remembering things. We would read a book together, but she couldn't remember what happened in the beginning of it. She would repeat the same comments and ask the same questions. My patience was growing thin. She was different. It was hard to imagine that this was the same little girl who was running through our front yard a week earlier, cracking jokes. I kept thinking that this was temporary. This had to be temporary because we couldn't go on living like this if it was permanent. Dave brought up her memory problem one night and I just shook my head. "No. It has to get better," was my only response to him.

We followed up with the neurologist a week later and I relayed that her memory seemed to be gone. He did some cursory testing and couldn't believe it was from the surgery. He couldn't understand how this didn't show up on her functional MRI—some name recall and comprehension testing had been done. Regardless, it happened, and I wanted to know how long it was going to last. He couldn't say nor would he predict. The doctor just hoped, like we did, that Emily's memory would gradually get better.

By now I knew I just had to take things day by day. I should have known that we could never predict the future with Emily. Ryan was now one and a half years old. It had been two years since we thought this was all behind us. This was supposed to be his time. Instead we were still wrapped up in all of Emily's medical stuff. Little did I know that it was just the beginning of the biggest battle yet.

Second grade started shortly after Emily recovered from this surgery. Her short-term memory was compromised, but her good spirit and all other functions sprang back. Unfortunately, so did her seizures. Granted, she wasn't having as many and she hadn't lost control of her bladder during a seizure, but the seizure activity was there. The same aide from first grade met Emily and me at the doors on the first day of second grade, and I realized then how much Emily needed her. Emily could now easily get disoriented since she couldn't remember where her new classroom was or even the new teacher's name (she could remember all her past teachers—that was a long-term memory). Anything new was difficult for her. Yet it didn't frustrate her. She took this setback like she did everything else in her life, with matter-of-factness and a "so what" attitude. She could only use one hand. So what? She had to wear a brace on her leg. So what? She had seizures. So what? She still played, had friends, went to school, read and did math. This, in turn, made parenting her so much easier than it could have been. She wasn't upset about it; why should we be?

In addition to the slew of regular doctor appointments Emily had, she still endured MRIs of her brain every three months to make sure the tumor wasn't growing. I still went through the emotions I did when Emily first started this routine. Worry about the tumor growing was always on my mind, but it would slowly creep forward during the days leading up to the MRI. Worry was still there even though the tumor hadn't grown in more than two years. And the routine MRI that occurred just three months after Emily's epilepsy surgery proved that I couldn't let my guard down.

After the scan, the oncologist came into the room that Emily and I were sitting in and announced, "I'm afraid the tumor is growing." I didn't respond. No matter how often I had heard that awful statement, it still froze me. The nurse practitioner popped in and took Emily to the other room to play while the doctor and I talked. We had to do something, he relayed, but we were out of chemotherapy options. She had already tried the therapies available for that type of tumor, and they had all failed. There was no reason to believe trying again would bring different results. She already had radiation, and that was typically done once. He was going to refer us to the surgeon to see if surgery was an option. But he warned that too many surgeries posed their own danger. At that point, I asked, "Are we allowed to say no if we don't want to do surgery?"

It was embarrassing not knowing our own rights with our child. Dave and I had talked over the last few months about how much more quality of life meant to us than the length of life. This was, of course, in regard to Emily's seizure activity and failing memory. And now she was faced with potentially enduring another invasive brain surgery that had the possibility of doing more harm. After all, we knew the risks from all those consent forms we had signed over the years.

He said, "You can absolutely refuse surgery. If you don't like the risks involved, you say no." Emily really had exhausted treatment options at this point, but we would meet with the surgeon to see what he thought. And although knowing we held the power to consent to surgery should have brought relief, it didn't. Her future was in our hands now.

I drove home that afternoon in a daze. I could no longer think of the future. I could only think of that minute and then the next minute; even the next day was too far. I was going to go home and tell Dave. That's how far my thoughts took me. And when I got home, I told him what the doctor said.

"What do you think about surgery again?" I asked.

He was silent for several minutes before stating, "I don't want to do anything that would damage her cognitive functions. A physical disability doesn't matter; she can overcome that. But for her to lose her cognitive abilities.... It's already hard dealing with the memory problems."

"I completely agree. We're allowed to refuse surgery if we don't want to do it." And that was it. We had to endure the rest of the night not knowing the fate of Emily's future. We went through the motions of the evening like robots—make dinner, bathe kids, bedtime.

The next day both Dave and I met with the surgeon. As he had been with surgeries past, he was quite confident that he could remove one of the tumors (there were three now) and debulk the others. Dave relayed our concerns, saying we didn't want to do surgery if her cognitive abilities were going to be impaired. The surgeon didn't think that would be an issue. And just like that, surgery was scheduled for the end of the week.

That Friday, I said goodbye to Ryan and Dave. Dave didn't want to deal with the hospital, and I was happy to not deal with his stress and to have him home taking care of Ryan. I spent the few days leading up to the surgery on autopilot. I wrapped up things at work in order to be off for a week, packed bags for both Emily and me for a week at the hospital and got everything in order for Ryan and Dave to be home on their own for a week. There wasn't enough time to feel the gravity of the situation—the fact that Emily was enduring yet another major brain surgery. That the tumor had grown again. We concentrated on the fact that we'd be home by next week and things could once again finally be back to normal.

Emily hopped into the car and I drove the 40 minutes to the hospital. Here we were *again* on our way to Children's Hospital for *another* craniotomy to debulk this tumor. I felt like Norm from *Cheers* as I walked the halls when we arrived ... *what are you guys doing here? Why is Emily back? Good luck with everything!* We ran into nurses, doctors, occupational therapists and physical therapists. The social workers even knew us by now and stopped to chat.

We went straight to the fifth floor for Emily to receive her antibiotics. After that, Emily was given her "frequent flyer" medication and then wheeled into the operating room. I held her hand while the gas made her fall asleep and kissed her goodbye before a nurse escorted me out of the surgical area. A few minutes later, I was down in the waiting room sipping coffee with my parents when a surgical resident came running down the hall, shoving papers at me. "I forgot to have you sign the consent forms!" No wonder this time seemed easier. No one reminded me of the risks minutes before kissing her goodbye.

The phone calls were coming every hour, and every hour I breathed easier after hearing that Emily was doing great. Jeff, Mike and Kim showed up and we sat in our corner of the waiting room for the remainder of the day. I would call home to Dave after every phone call I received from the operating room to keep him apprised of Emily's progress and so I could hear how Ryan was doing.

Ryan was now 18 months old and a full-on toddler. He loved to walk around in snow boots regardless of the temperature. He also loved his pacifiers—typically one in his mouth and an extra one in his hand. His other hand usually dragged a toy of some sort—a plastic golf club, a plastic truck, or a superhero figure. He was proving to be all *boy*, even though he also loved to wear Emily's headbands and play with her toys. We would often find him lying on the floor, wearing Emily's pink headband, playing with his toy trucks and cars. We thought it was so neat to watch him push Emily's baby doll around the house in the baby stroller too. What a great dad he'll be someday! Until we watched him flip the stroller over, baby doll flying, and sit and spin the wheels of the stroller, just fascinated with how the wheels worked—without a care that the doll was missing. So much for my progressive son.

By this age, Emily had quite a few words, speaking in sentences, even, but Ryan was content with "Mama," "Dada," "Emmy," "baba" (bottle) and "no." The essentials. He had no need for more words as Emily would often talk for him and usually over him. Having a bossy big sister meant that you had a lot of patience and also that you were waited on hand and foot. Emily loved being my helper when she could. There were other times, though, usually when she was tired, which was becoming more and more often the case, that Emily wanted nothing to do with her little brother. She would be lounging on the couch playing her Leapster or watching TV and Ryan would toddle over for some attention. Instead she would roll over so her back was to him with a look of sisterly annoyance on her face. At this point, Ryan would give an impish grin and try to poke or prod her. She would then grunt at him or yell for me to take him away.

It wasn't hard to see that these two had a different sibling relationship. There was the six-year age difference along with the fact that Emily had physical differences and significant medical needs which made their interactions look different than the siblings we saw around us. Ryan was gentle with her from the get-go. We don't know if it was just his nature or if he understood she was a bit more fragile than most kids. Emily, though, liked to instigate some shenanigans. For the longest time, Ryan would cry when he was buckled into his rear -facing car seat. Not right away—only after we were driving for a few minutes. I finally caught Emily pointing her finger at his face, but not quite touching him. He didn't stop crying until she pulled her hand away. After busting Emily, with her giving us the *But I'm not touching him!* excuse, she stopped, and he didn't have those crying fits anymore. Moments of these normal sibling fights perhaps would make other moms frustrated. Instead they made me smile. It was a hint of normalcy.

And now I was sitting in a hospital waiting room while Emily was having her eighth brain surgery and Dave and Ryan were at home trying to have a regular day. Our neighborhood had changed; most of our good friends had moved away, but those who were around stopped by that day to check on Dave and get the progress reports on Emily.

The surgeon finally came into the waiting room, eight hours later, to say that all went well. He was able to remove significant portions of the tumors. He relayed that she was still heavily medicated but content in the ICU. I was so tired of this routine. Again, I just nodded and waited for the nurse to escort me to the ICU so I could see Emily myself. About 15 minutes later the nurse took me to the ICU. Em looked so peaceful. She still had a breathing tube in and IVs in both arms, chest monitors hooked up and a blood pressure cuff on her leg. The white turban bandage was on her head while she lay on the bed asleep—no more crib for her now that she was seven years old.

That evening the ICU nurses and doctor removed her breathing tube and she continued to breathe fine. Usually she would be awake by now, cranky and asking for juice, but she was still asleep. I called home to Dave to say that she was comfortable and not even awake. It probably was not worth it to get childcare that night for him to come in. So he stayed home with Ryan, and soon my parents, Jeff, Mike and Kim left for their homes. I sat in the brightly-lit room with machines sounding, our nurse fleeting in and out every 15 minutes, and Emily still not stirring. Soon I drifted off to sleep and didn't wake again until morning. I had slept through it all. Emily had too. She was still sleeping soundly. The nurse reported that she hadn't made a peep all night.

I called home to Dave to check in on him and Ryan. It was a typical night and morning for them, and he was glad to hear that Emily was so comfortable. But we both talked about how odd it was that she hadn't stirred. I sat on Emily's bed next to her, in between all the cords and lines, and gently nudged her. I called her name and stroked her cheek asking if she was ready for some juice. She moved her head and adjusted a bit but didn't wake up. She was moving—it wasn't like she was paralyzed which was the fear a few surgeries ago. It was just strange she hadn't woken up. This concern lingered all day as people came in and out to visit Emily, still sleeping soundly even through our gentle nudgings.

Doctors in the ICU didn't form an opinion one way or the other on her condition. All her vitals were stable, and she was breathing on her own and moving. She was older now, I kept telling myself. It takes longer to recover from injuries the older you are. My mom and dad sat with me, watching Emily sleep, but unable to hide their concern. The doctors don't seem to be worried. "Let's just be happy she's not uncomfortable" became my mantra.

Emily remained in the ICU for four days, still not conscious. At that point the doctors relayed that she no longer needed the ICU. All her vital signs were all good, she was just sleepy. I, on the other hand, was worried. This was not how she reacted after any of her previous surgeries. I was anxious for her to wake up. After all, I knew we couldn't go home until she was up, eating and walking. My plan to be home within a day or two, back to normal as a complete family, didn't look promising.

Dave had been coming in to visit Emily daily and I would go home to spend time with Ryan and to shower. I didn't know how much longer we could keep up that routine. When I was gone, I was scared she was going to wake up and want her mom. It was also getting harder and harder to say goodbye to Ryan every afternoon, and frankly, I didn't know how much longer Dave had it in him had to be a single dad—a single dad who was taking care of a toddler at home while worrying about his daughter in the ICU.

On the fifth day, we went directly to a private room on the fifth floor. The damn fifth floor again. The nurses, always so cheerful, welcomed us into the room and we got settled. That evening Elisa came after work to visit just as the nurses were doing Emily's vital signs routine. Emily had spiked a fever and her blood pressure shot up to an alarming level. The stress in the room was palpable as the nurse paged the doctor and I stood over Emily holding her hand with my trembling hand. Within minutes we were wheeled down to radiology for a CT scan. I could feel my stomach bloating by the second as the stress radiated through my body. When we got to the CT scan machine, the techs asked not once but *twice* if I was pregnant to make sure I could be in the room with Emily. "No!" I finally shouted. "Just a little stress bloat!" That was enough to ease the tension in the room as Elisa couldn't contain her laughter at my reaction.

The CT scan didn't show anything different that could be causing the fever or rise in blood pressure. Back in the room, medicines were administered and the fever went down slightly, as did her blood pressure. The surgeon came in and was alarmed at Emily's vitals. He ordered an MRI to be done first thing in the morning. I made my phone calls home to let everyone know that we were now out of the ICU, but no, Emily had still not woken up. I left a voicemail for my supervisor stating that I would not be back at work next week like originally planned and that I would call him within a day to talk further. That night I went to sleep on the window seat cushion next to Emily's bed, hopeful for answers from the morning's scheduled MRI.

At 6 a.m. we went down for the MRI and, like usual, I used that time to grab coffee and some breakfast from the hospital cafeteria. When she was done with the scan we went back to the room and met the surgeon there. He had printed images of the MRI and held them up to the light for me to see. "Here, see this? It's a cerebral infarction," the surgeon went on, "this explains Emily's condition."

"What does that mean?" I asked.

"She had a stroke leaving her in this coma."

≈ 11 ≈

Home Away from Home

I accepted the news that Emily suffered a stroke with a quick nod of my head and asked no questions. I didn't comprehend what that meant for Emily, and I didn't know what to ask to get a better understanding. I later wished I had asked what specifically caused the stroke. How long would she be in a coma? What would her recovery look like? Does this mean she lost any functioning? Instead I was left in the dark feeling blindsided, unable to form any thoughts. My visit with the surgeon lasted no more than five minutes, and then it was just Emily and me alone in the room. And Emily was still unconscious.

I called Dave. "The surgeon was just here. He said Emily had a stroke."

"What? What does that mean?"

"I don't know. That's all I know. Can you come in with Ryan?" I needed them right now in my arms. "I can visit with him here now that Emily's out of the ICU."

I paced inside Emily's room the rest of the morning, checking out the doorway every few minutes to see if Dave and Ryan were there yet. Finally, I saw them coming down the hall. Ryan had a pacifier in his mouth, one hand was holding Dave's hand, the other hand holding another pacifier, and he wore Emily's purple headband, *Star Trek*–style, over his eyes. I couldn't help but laugh at the sight of him and he smiled over his pacifier. I came out of the room, picked him up, walked toward Emily's room and said, "Let's go see Emmy!" With that he giggled.

We got to the room where Emily lay in bed, oxygen tubes in her nose, chest monitors attached to her chest, IVs in both arms with pumps attached, and a blood pressure cuff on her leg. She still had a turban made of bandages on her head and her left eye was swollen. Ryan looked at her and cried. I put him down because he started kicking. I kneeled next to him repeating, "It's okay, buddy, she's okay." He cried harder and harder and ran out the door. I caught up to him and walked with him back to the room, but he stopped in the doorway and screamed.

"I'm taking him home," Dave said and quickly left with him.

Just as they left, leaving me alone in the room with Emily, feeling like I just got sucker punched, the oncologist and his nurse practitioner, who had been caring for Emily since her diagnosis, came in. I had to shove away the pain I felt from not being able to hold my son as I faced the doctor. I told them what the surgeon said. The oncologist put his head down and mumbled, "Shit. He [the surgeon] should never have gone in again." The oncologist was weary of the amount of surgeries Emily had on her brain, perhaps knowing that eventually this would happen. Even though I should have been angry, too, I wanted to come to the surgeon's defense. *He was just trying to save my daughter's life*, I would have said, if I had the ability to form words. Instead, reality was sinking in. Emily was in a coma. Ryan was scared. Dave was angry. My life, as I knew it, was flipped completely upside down.

The nurse practitioner asked, "Are you okay?" I shrugged. She asked, "How's Dave? Is he here?"

"No," I started crying, not being able to contain my hurt anymore. "He just came here with Ryan, but Ryan ... he didn't want to come in the room."

The nurse practitioner started crying, reminding me that medical professionals are human too, hugged me, and said she was sorry. The doctor led her out of the room and they walked away.

My parents came to see us that afternoon. My brother, Jeff, also stopped by after work. We all took turns trying to wake Emily up, yet never wanting her to be uncomfortable. We sat on my window seat bed and the recliner chair in the room and stared at the small, broken form of Emily. I couldn't make small talk, and neither could anyone else. The cheery nurses came into the room every few hours to check Emily's vitals and adjust her IV pump. That night, I went to sleep on the window seat not realizing I would be sleeping on that cushion every night for the next two months.

The next day, Dave dropped Ryan off at my parents' house before coming to visit Emily. While he was there, I was able to take a shower and eat a full meal in the cafeteria. "Why don't you come home tonight?" he asked.

"I can't leave her," I simply replied.

"She's not even awake."

"Exactly. What if she wakes up and I'm not here? No, I can't leave."

"The nurses are here checking on her all the time." Dave was pleading now. "And what about Ryan?"

"I'll go home while you're here tomorrow and spend the afternoon with him. I'll be able to do some laundry and repack my bag too."

"What am I supposed to do about work—I'm out of vacation days. What are we going to do with Ryan?"

Frustrated with him, with everything, I responded, "I *don't* know. I *can't* leave Emily. I don't know how long she's going to be here."

I was on the verge of tears but couldn't cry. I was too numb to feel anything. The slow realization of not knowing Emily's future, and ours, was suffocating. We stopped talking about it and he tried waking Emily. He talked loudly to her, stroking her face, even shook the bed. Still no reaction from her.

That night my mom, with true mother's intuition, called to say that she and my dad would watch Ryan so that Dave could go back to work. She remembered that Dave had already taken two weeks off work for Emily's surgery. They found a crib and highchair to use so that Ryan could spend the night at their house on Dave's long workdays. On Dave's days off, Ryan would go back home to Dave. That news brought a big sigh of relief. At least Dave could get back to work—some semblance of routine for him and a break from the baby.

I called my supervisor the next morning, explained Emily's situation, and said I didn't know when I could go back to work. Again, my supervisor said, without hesitation, that I could take family medical leave—I had up to 12 weeks to use. One more thing I didn't have to worry about. I may not have a paycheck coming in, but I had a job to go back to when I was ready. I called Emily's elementary school and updated them on her situation and said she wouldn't be back to school for a few weeks.

That same morning Dave came in to see Emily with Ryan in tow. I met them in the downstairs lobby so that I could take Ryan home with me without him having to see Emily in her current state. At home I did my laundry and took a long shower. Then I played in the backyard for hours with Ryan. We kicked the soccer ball, he hit the plastic ball off the tee, and we hunted for sticks. I soaked him and the sunshine in but had a nagging ache in the back of my head thinking of Emily lying unconscious in the hospital. When Ryan went down for the night, I called Elisa to come over and watch him so I could go back to the hospital and relieve Dave. When Dave got home, he relieved Elisa of the babysitting duty. The amount of planning involved just so I could be there for my kids felt overwhelming.

The following week, Mike stopped by after work. He asked if I had voted. I was a big news watcher and usually followed politics, but I looked at him with disgust. "No, of course I haven't voted. I've been living in a hospital!" I didn't even realize it was Election Day. I was so angry that the world was still spinning and that people were going on with their lives. *Emily hasn't woken up yet! She had a stroke!* I wanted to shout to the world. How could people be living their lives when mine had come to a screeching halt?

That night Emily fluttered her eyes open. I ran to her bedside and immediately started talking, "Hi, sweetie! How are you feeling? Do you want some juice?" I never got a response. She just looked at me with her big blue eyes.

Then the pleading and begging started. "Hey, sweetie. Em. Emmy. Emily. Mommy's here," I said.

Still no response, just a blank look. I called the nurse to the room. She repeated the same questions I had just asked and got the same non-response. Emily stayed awake for about 10 minutes and then went back to sleep. The 10 minutes of her eyes being open gave me all the hope I needed, though. It was a step forward. She was in there.

This pattern continued all the next day. She would open her eyes but not speak. She would also not move. She couldn't sit up on her own. She couldn't eat on her own. She now had a feeding tube down her nose for nutrition. The catheter was removed and now she wore diapers. Her oxygen levels would sometimes dip too low and she would require an oxygen mask. My almost-eight-year-old daughter, who just weeks earlier skipped through the halls of second grade talking non-stop, was now confined to a bed unable to do the most basic functions. It was almost worse that she laid there with her eyes open and not able to talk.

Emily's condition did not change. She was in a semi-comatose state, awake but not functioning. Every morning I prayed, *Please let this be the day that she asks for juice.* The days suddenly turned into weeks. It was like walking through a desert where the scenery doesn't change, and you don't know if it ever will. If it does, you don't know what the new landscape is going to look like—a terrifying feeling. I stared and begged and pled with her to wake up and talk, day in and day out, in that tiny room that housed a bed, a bathroom, a recliner, and a window seat. At night, exhausted from my pleading, I laid on the window seat and slept for two hours at a time—in between the nurses coming in to take her vitals. I was awakened by the morning rounds every day only to sit in that room and stare at her all day again.

I only saw Ryan every few days now, the coordination to visit him along with my primal instincts to not leave Emily proving difficult to navigate. Every night I slept on the window seat cushion. Every morning I would brush my teeth and wash my face in Emily's bathroom. I changed out of my sweatpants into a pair of jeans and put on a new sweatshirt. I waited until after morning rounds before walking down the hall to get a cup of coffee—alerting a nurse that I was leaving the room for a few minutes. I would try to wait for a visitor to stay with Emily before running down to the cafeteria to grab breakfast, lunch, or dinner to go. If I couldn't make it to the cafeteria, I ate the snacks that friends were bringing me ... an eclectic assortment of various chocolates, almonds, and popcorn. I ran down the hallway to the parent coffee pot every few hours to feed my addiction that helped me be alert. I took a shower every few days, either at home when I got a visit in with Ryan or in the Ronald McDonald parent room.

The evenings, after visitors left, were spent on the phone with Dave. Most nights, after the daily rundown, the calls turned dark. Dave asked why I was still sleeping at the hospital and I questioned him for even asking me. He understood, he would say, but this was no life. He wanted me home with him and Ryan. My mom and Kim offered to stay with Emily, but I never let them. I just couldn't leave her, and this hurt Dave.

Sometimes we talked about Emily's future, guessing at what it would look like. *What if this was it?* We confessed to each other during these late-night calls that we would have preferred she died than to live in this vegetative state. The little girl lying in the bed, not talking, joking, laughing or even sitting up … that was not our Emily. After this confession, I cried over the guilt I suddenly felt. How could a mother think that of her child?

There were phone calls when Dave screamed and I cried. There were times when Dave admitted he wanted to leave us and I told him to go ahead. He didn't leave, of course. He was too responsible and had too much love for Emily and Ryan, and perhaps me, to leave. At this point, I didn't know if our relationship would survive. I also didn't care. Obviously, I loved him—his humor, his heart, his intellect—I just didn't have what it took to keep us going at that time. I had only enough energy to concentrate on Emily getting better and to try to get Ryan out of this unscathed.

Regardless of how each phone call ended the previous night, we talked the next day. We didn't revisit the conversations we had in the dark evenings. We talked with each other like we usually did, with humor. Dave joked about getting used to eating pizza for dinner night after night, and I joked about the fact that I missed vegetables after eating fried hospital food day after day. We laughed that our credit card bill was the lowest it had ever been with me being trapped in the hospital and unable to shop.

We called Dave's parents in Connecticut every few days to update them on Emily's condition. Tammy, Dave's older sister, checked in regularly. Tammy was incredibly close to Emily despite the miles between them. She was an avid skier and flew to Colorado often, staying with us during her visits.

During one phone call early in Emily's stay on the fifth floor, Tammy announced, "I'm looking at tickets to fly out for the weekend. I'm going to see if Mom will come with me." I told her she didn't need to—she worked full-time and had a two-year-old *and* one-year-old twin boys. But she said, "I need to. I need to see Emily and my brother." Tammy arranged for her mother-in-law to help her husband take care of the kids and got her mom, who was hesitant to travel, to fly to Colorado with her.

My dad picked them up from the airport and brought them straight to the hospital where they stayed for the day, sitting by Emily's side. Dave came in to get them that evening and they stayed with Dave and Ryan for the weekend, coming to the hospital for a few hours at a time. I thought for sure once my mother-in-law saw our situation with her own eyes she would offer to stay longer. She was always so giving of her time taking care of Dave's nieces and nephews, I was sure she would stay to help us. I even admitted to her how much Dave and I could use her support—both emotionally and logistically. But she ended up going home at the end of the weekend. She said she had her job to get back to and was also baby-sitting Dave's younger sister's son during the day. The rejection and disappointment I felt when she left hit me like a ton of bricks. As my father drove them back to the airport, I called my mom and cried. I just sobbed and sobbed and sobbed. My mother, on the other end of the phone, kept repeating, "Let it out. It's okay to cry. Let it all out." I believe it was the first time my mother had heard me cry since the day Emily was diagnosed with a brain tumor.

During the third week of our stay, my friend Sandy came to visit bearing a gift—a coffee maker for the room. I practically kissed her on the lips for this ingenious gift. It never occurred to me to get one, probably because it wasn't allowed. And although I was a rule-follower by nature, I had no problem plugging that baby in and placing it on the little table next to the window seat. I just pulled the curtain around it to hide it from the nurses and doctors. They all knew I had one, of course, because the nurses always commented that my room always smelled so wonderful as they watched me drink coffee from my personal mug. No one ever asked me to unplug it and I was able to have coffee first thing in the morning and any time I wanted after that.

Thanksgiving week arrived and Emily was still in her semi-comatose state although now she occasionally screamed. The shouts were random and often short-lived. She would also, amazingly enough, engage in games of thumb wars. Mike realized, one day while holding her hand, that her thumb was moving. He went into a game.... *One, two, three, four, I declare a thumb war!* We then watched with wide eyes as she wrapped her thumb around Mike's and pegged him. And then she smiled. My little fighter was in there.

Phone calls were gleefully made to everyone we knew. And every visitor after that day played Thumb War with Emily. I talked with Emily more and more as well. Up until this point, I read her books and she was my sounding board as I talked to myself through-out the day. But now she would smile at certain parts of the book which made me work harder to make her grin. I would read a story about a frog and exclaim, in an exaggerated voice, "Ew! Gross, frogs! Why are you making me read about frogs? Are you trying to creep me out?" She would then smile.

The day before Thanksgiving my friend Sandy called and said, "I'm going to sit with Emily tomorrow while you have dinner with your family."

"No, you're not. Have dinner with your own kid and family. You've done plenty," I said as I sipped coffee made from my personal coffee maker.

"I wasn't asking. What time is your family planning dinner? If I came at 1 o'clock would that work?"

"What about your family?" I countered.

"They're having dinner with my in-laws. They'll be fine," she said.

The next day Sandy arrived all bundled up from the cold weather outside, holding the newspaper with all the Black Friday ads, and sat down on the recliner. All she said was, "Hi, Em! I'm going to hang out with you today, kiddo." Then she looked at me and said, "Okay, go. Enjoy, take a long shower, eat, and don't rush."

Sandy and I knew each other because her son and Emily were friends and had been in school together since their first year of pre-school. I always enjoyed her company and hung out with her a few times socially, but she wasn't part of my circle of friends I saw or talked with daily. Yet, Sandy seemed to easily step in and be there for me. Perhaps she understood more than most people because she grew up with a sister who had medical and cognitive disabilities and Sandy was one of her primary caregivers. She, of all people, knew what we were up against.

That Thanksgiving I sat at Jeff's dining room table with the rest of my family. Ryan sat on my lap and ate off my plate and I smiled.

This was family. My friends coming to the hospital on a constant basis became my family. On this day of thanks, I truly understood the meaning of family and what to be grateful for. And as grateful as I was to be sitting at that table, I was anxious to get back to the hospital, unable to shake the image of Emily lying in bed, not here with us.

Now that Emily was awake more and more during the day and engaging, somewhat, with her surroundings, she started work with a physical therapist. She would be wheeled down the hall to the gym where a therapist worked on basic skills like sitting up. They placed her in a standing position to get weight on her legs. They lifted her arm and had her hold it in the air. Emily screamed quite a few times during these therapy sessions and would go right to sleep afterward, exhausted.

During one of the initial therapy sessions the physical therapist said it was time to order a wheelchair for her. A slow realization of what our new normal would look like came over me. A wheelchair. She took all of Emily's measurements and showed me all the parts of the chair she was ordering that would best meet Emily's needs. She then asked Emily what color chair she wanted, and I responded that yellow was her favorite color. Like everything during that hospital stay, though, I could only think about that day and the next day. I couldn't think about next week, month or year.

The occupational therapist visited Emily in her room on a regular basis. The first time she came into the room she announced, "Hi, Emily, it's time to get dressed." I looked at her like she was crazy. We obviously weren't going anywhere, and the hospital gown worked well with all the lines and cords. As she struggled to get Emily's arm out of the gown, I shook my head and said, "Stop. There isn't a reason to get her dressed. Shouldn't we be concentrating on getting her to sit up or something basic like that?" The therapist explained that some movements are rote—so engrained in our daily lives that muscle memory takes over. And then I watched as Emily slipped her arm through her shirt. Well, I'll be damned. It was another moment of hope for me.

My parents were slowly getting used to living with an active toddler again. Early wake-up calls, diaper changes, temper tantrums and time-outs were now a part of their retirement. They let me know, though, that they were enjoying the time with Ryan, as exhausted as they were. Ryan was still full of cuddles and hugs and my mom especially loved the chunks on his thighs. Her "little Michelin Man," she would call him. My dad, to this day, whispers, "Hot, hot" with emphasis on the "t" every time the stove burner is on, imitating Ryan during his stay with them. At a minimum, Ryan ended up providing my parents a great distraction.

After week six in the hospital, all my conversations with the doctors revolved around going home. As overwhelming as it was to think about taking care of Emily at home, I couldn't think of staying in the hospital any longer. I was at my breaking point. We needed to be a complete family again. I was tired of the separate lives. My evening phone calls with Dave were getting darker and darker. But mostly, I needed to be with Ryan as much as I needed to be with Emily. I couldn't stand the separation anymore.

The doctors told us Emily needed a G-tube inserted in order to think about going home. This was a feeding tube implanted directly into her stomach, with a plug on the outside of her abdomen to which the IV line with formula would attach. It was a better alternative to the feeding tube in her nose which kept getting displaced. There was a problem, though. She would need surgery, with full anesthesia, to have it implanted. The thought of her enduring another surgery immediately made Dave say no. And I couldn't schedule the surgery until he was on board, which didn't happen for another day when he finally agreed it was worth the risk. By the end of the week, the procedure was conducted, and I was trained how to do the feedings myself.

A few days later her bright yellow wheelchair arrived at the hospital. It was heavy and had a lot of parts, but it also meant we were another step closer to going home. Dave went to the car dealership and quickly traded his Mustang for a minivan. He took a good amount of ribbing from the guys at the dealership for making that trade, not believing anyone would give up a sports car for a minivan. Dave finally admitted to the salesman, "We need a vehicle that could fit a wheelchair."

A week before Christmas we received our discharge papers. It was with great excitement, and anxiety, that I signed them. I packed all my bags and the nurses got Emily buckled into her new wheelchair. Medical supplies, like an IV pump, formula, and diapers, were ordered and already sent to the house. The nurses walked with us to the parking garage for a big send-off, and Dave drove us home in the new minivan. Once home, he carried Emily, now just a month shy of eight years old, from the car to the reclining chair in our family room, his eyes watering when Emily tried talking and only indistinct noise came out. I took a deep breath and walked into our home, having no idea how we were going to do this.

When I told my parents that we were going home, they were flabbergasted. My mom immediately asked, "Are you going to hire a nurse?"

"No, I'm going to take care of her."

"How? What about a rehabilitation facility? Wouldn't she be better off going there?" she persisted.

"No, she's going home," I replied with annoyance. I couldn't understand why she didn't think Emily should be home with me, Dave and Ryan. But when I walked through the door and it was just us, with no nursing staff and no hospital equipment, I came to fully realize her concern.

⇒ 12 ⇐

Home Sweet Home

Dave got Emily settled in the beige recliner that once was considered his chair. He put a bed pillow behind her head, a waterproof "chuck" on the seat of the chair, and had the legs extended up. I quickly got the IV pump set up next to the chair to get ready for a feeding and changed her diaper. Once all of our bags were brought in and put away, I called my parents and asked them to bring Ryan home. It was time to be a family again.

My mom and dad walked straight into the house 30 minutes later, Ryan strolling in front of them. As soon as Ryan saw Emily sitting in the reclining chair, he clapped. He giggled, smiling so big his pacifier fell out of his mouth, and clapped some more. Dave swooped him up and placed him next to Emily in the chair. They both sat silently, side by side, with smiles on their faces. I watched them and felt slightly better about my decision to push for her to go home. My parents, teary at Ryan's reaction, left for their home after giving Emily lots of kisses and squeezes. And then it was just us.

That night we ate dinner together—a casserole someone had brought over. Dave and I sat at the kitchen table, Ryan in his highchair, and Emily in her chair in the family room which was open to the kitchen. We were finally together. I gave Ryan a bath and put him to bed shortly after dinner. Such a normal thing to do, but I felt so privileged to be able to do it. Dave sat on the couch next to Emily who was dozing in and out of consciousness, and watched TV. I came downstairs, after somehow getting through most of the day at home, and asked Dave, "How are we going to do this?"

He responded, "We'll just bring the IV pole upstairs and I'll carry Em to bed."

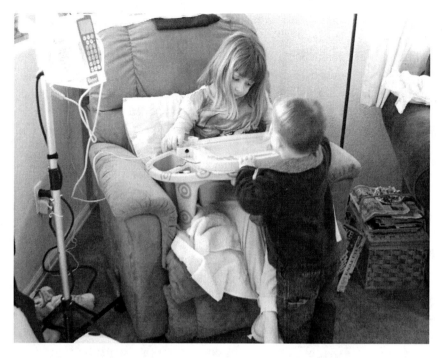

Emily, age eight, at home recovering from a stroke, with Ryan bringing her toys.

I had meant the more general *How are we going to take care of this incredibly disabled child and an active toddler?* but he took it to mean *How are we going to get through tonight?* I didn't clarify my meaning because I realized there was no answer. I needed to get back to thinking only of today and tomorrow.

As promised, Dave carried Emily up the flight of stairs to her bedroom. We made a big fuss about being back in her own bed, but Emily just stared at us with a smile. The doctors had warned us that her sleep cycle was probably off and prescribed her a sleep aid that I put in a syringe and administered through her G-tube. Once that was in, along with all her seizure meds, I hooked her formula up to the IV lines and attached that to her feeding tube. She was to receive a slow rate of formula at bedtime for about six hours. I set my alarm for six hours later, afraid I wouldn't hear the pump beeping ... immune to it after sleeping in a hospital for so long. And for the first time in almost two months, I slept in a real bed. My own bed, next to my husband, both my kids sleeping in their own rooms down the hall from me.

At 3 a.m. my alarm went off and I shut off the already-beeping IV pump. Emily was still sleeping as I unhooked the IV line from her G-tube. I went back to bed and quickly fell back to sleep awaiting Ryan to wake me up next. Without fail, he woke me up three hours later. And just like giving him a bath the night before, instead of annoyed, I was grateful for something so normal, to be able to be the one to greet him in the morning. On my way to bring him downstairs, I peeked in on Emily and noticed she was awake. I quickly got Ryan settled so that I could wake Dave up to have him carry Emily down. Without comment, Dave lifted Emily out of bed and carried her down the flight of stairs to the recliner in the family room. He then, again without comment, turned around and went straight back to bed.

That first full day at home was exhilarating and exhausting. I was thrilled to be home again, not having the stress of coordinating visits to and from the hospital. I was no longer worried about how Dave or my parents were handling their duties with Ryan. I would gladly juggle two kids in diapers, two kids not quite verbal, a constant inventory of medical supplies, and dealing with a feeding tube that was a bit finicky than be separated again. I was also chained to my house. I couldn't just throw the kids in the car and run to the grocery store if I needed something.

The parents at Emily's school put together a meal train providing us dinner every night for several months. At about 4 every other afternoon there would be a knock on our front door letting us know that dinner was sitting in a cooler, or more often than not that winter, placed on top of the snow drift outside our door. Colleagues of mine from work also put together a large gift basket, including, among other things, a gift certificate for a housecleaner visit. These gifts proved to be a necessity I didn't realize I needed. Most of our time was spent managing Emily—her meds, her diapers, moving her, and trying to stimulate her—and any leftover time was spent in an attempt to make up for lost time with Ryan. So when we ate dinner, we thought of the family who thought of us that day and were thankful to be surrounded by such a caring group. When I played trucks with Ryan instead of dusting and vacuuming, I thought of my coworkers and felt thankful for their generosity.

That second night at home, Dave carried Emily up the flight

of stairs to her bed. I hooked her feeding tube up again for the night-time feeding, and we went off to watch TV in bed. But an hour later, the IV pump beeped. There was a kink in the line. I fixed it and proudly announced to Dave that I was able to troubleshoot my first IV pump error. "I could so be a nurse!" I proclaimed, bragging about my new skills. But when I went in at 3 a.m. to turn the pump off after the feeding ended, the distinct smell of formula stopped me at the door. Emily was lying in a pool of creamy, thick formula that had been dripping, at a slow rate, for five hours on top of her abdomen instead of into her stomach. She was drenched and upset and probably had been for hours, with no way of letting me know, while I slept soundly in my bed in the next room. With gut-wrenching guilt, I woke Dave up to help me. I got her undressed and he carried her to the bathtub, where I gave her my first solo bath. This poor child was dependent on me and I blew it.

Dave stripped her bed and made it again, then carried Emily back to bed from the bathtub. Less than two hours later, at 5 a.m., his alarm went off so that he could go to work. Once Dave was showered and dressed, he woke me up and carried Emily downstairs. He then announced, with coffee cup in hand, "Bye, I get to go to work now. I mean, I have to go to work now." I laughed. Yes, we both knew that being at work felt like a day at the spa compared to being at home.

Christmas came and went that year like it was just another day. Emily, of course, didn't run into our room announcing that Santa came, begging us to wake up so we could open presents. Ryan was still too young to understand the significance of the day. Instead, he woke up at his typical 6 o'clock and Dave carried Emily downstairs. If it weren't for the overabundance of gifts from our family tripping us everywhere, it would have been a regular day.

I didn't step foot in a single store leading up to Christmas that year and that was just fine with me. I shopped online for small gifts for my nieces and nephews and bought a minimal number of toys for Emily and Ryan. It wasn't important. It truly, without a doubt, was not important. I never used to go overboard for the holidays like some people, but I did enjoy shopping for the kids and seeing their faces on Christmas morning. That year I didn't. The reality of Emily's life, how different our lives were now, along with a general feeling of remorse, had settled in. Besides, our families went over the top that year buying gifts for both kids.

After Christmas, life became routine. I started working limited hours from home giving my brain something else to think about. We stopped the nighttime feedings, giving Emily all her nutrients during the day, and giving us a full night of sleep. Emily no longer needed medicine to sleep at night; her internal clock had adjusted. I took Emily to physical, occupational, and speech therapy every week as well as to numerous follow-up appointments with all the specialists. The new minivan was getting a lot of miles put on it, and I developed a keen appreciation for nice weather and a hatred for snow, ice, rain and slush. There was nothing worse than pushing a wheelchair through a snow drift on a cracked sidewalk that hadn't been shoveled yet while also holding the hand of a toddler. Ryan and Emily learned a lot of new words that winter and none were appropriate for them to repeat.

Emily was slowly improving and becoming more alive. By the end of January, she could sit up. She would sit on the floor, with legs crossed and pillows scattered behind her to soften the blow for when she fell over, which she inevitably did, and play with Ryan. I often sat with them to build towers of blocks that both would take turns knocking over, then laugh hysterically. On a few occasions I had to stop Ryan from whipping a block at Emily and, conversely, I had to stop Emily from throwing it at Ryan, although I did applaud her throw attempt.

I used the same building blocks to quiz Emily. They had numbers and letters on them, and I would spread a handful out and ask her, "What letter does 'tiger' start with?" We high-fived for 20 minutes when she shakily pointed to the block with the letter T on it. I ignored the tugging at my throat when I thought how far she had slipped ... she used to be an advanced reader, and now she was working on the most basic skills. The speech therapist worked on vowel sounds with Emily as they were the easiest to form. After her first speech therapy session, Em mastered the sound "eee." So I interjected most days with questions like "What does your name start with?" She would proudly say, "Eeeeee."

Dave and I fell into a rhythm. We talked more now that we were living together and didn't have the unknown of how long Emily was going to be in the hospital or what life was going to be like when she got home. As ugly as it was, the unknown was uglier. We didn't go out during this time, either. Emily was still too fragile, and Dave had to be home in order to carry her upstairs at bedtime. He never complained about carrying her, other than stating she felt heavier and heavier each night. I suggested that she sleep in the chair downstairs with me on the couch, but he was insistent that this routine was fine. He brought her up to bed at 7:30 every night—the same time as Ryan. She was tired and nodding off by then, plus it gave Dave and me a break in the evenings. Sitting on the couch watching sitcoms was our nighttime norm and we would head to bed by 9, exhausted. Looking forward to those one and a half hours of uninterrupted time to ourselves, with my brain turned off as much as it could be, was what got me through most days.

On the weekends, Elisa would sometimes come over and hang out with us in the evenings. I understood, finally, that even though my life had drastically changed, the rest of the world moved on. And I wanted to be a part of that world. I wanted to laugh. I wanted to work. I wanted to socialize. My close friends understood this and nurtured it, even with my new set of limitations. I loved when someone came over, poured a drink, and bitched about their day. They didn't worry that I most likely had a worse day. I relished the fact that I could complain to my friends about my love handles as I ate chips and had a beer with them. I didn't feel judgment about my food choices or that that should be the least of my worries, the hum of the IV pump going as Emily sat next to us getting her nutrition through a hole in her stomach.

I rarely opened up about all the raw emotions I was going through, though, with my friends or family. I kept that for Dave. We still had many tear-filled evenings, but this time the anger wasn't directed at each other. We commiserated together. He felt everything I felt, and we were both comfortable screaming at the universe for the unfairness of it all. We had to say goodbye to our dreams that Emily would someday go off to college and become CEO of a company, putting her smart, confident bossiness to use. Instead, we were trying to come to grips with the reality that Emily might never leave our house. She might never get married. She might never have children. We danced the dance of being hopeful that she would recover and be her old self and yet, somehow, knowing that she wouldn't.

By the time Emily's eighth birthday rolled around she was awake most of the day and quick to smile. She tracked Ryan with her eyes, watched TV, and was actively engaged when anyone talked with her. We played about 15 games of Thumb War a day and she won them all. She also cheated, but I gave her a pass. She worked hard in speech therapy on speaking as well as eating. The therapist would put a frozen pea in her mouth and instruct her how to chew it and move it from one side of her mouth to the other. She had swallowed a few mushy food items, like a spoonful of mashed potatoes, at the therapist's office but still got all her nutrients from the formula through her G-tube. But on her birthday, surrounded by family instead of school friends, I gave her a bite of the chocolate birthday cake I had baked the day before. She reached for more and, since there were no issues swallowing it, I obliged. She ended up eating an entire slice. Chocolate proved to be her motivating factor once again.

Although I was chastised by the therapist after reporting this news to her, she did let me feed Emily more and more real food. We had to start with soft foods that did not require much energy to chew, like mashed potatoes and oatmeal. We could then move up to more and more solid food. Liquids were saved for last. They moved too fast in Emily's mouth, causing her to choke. By the end of March, she was only using the G-tube for liquids and medicines.

That spring, we enrolled Emily in a school program for homebound students that allowed for a teacher to come to our house a few mornings a week to work with Emily. The school district we were in provided this to us and let us know that this was the best option for Emily. When she started, Emily could still not talk. But as each week passed, she became more and more verbal. Emily would say a few one-word responses and soon was speaking in sentences. Long gone was my daughter who never seemed to stop talking. Now, she seemed to speak only when necessary with very labored and slow speech. Emily and the teacher would sit at our kitchen table and do worksheets and read books that the teacher had brought with her. We watched Emily go from practicing how to hold her pencil to writing her name. She also could read words at the same level she was at before the stroke. Emily was able to successfully complete her second grade at home with this homebound teacher, mostly due to how advanced she was when she started second grade.

Emily could also, by this time, walk if someone walked behind her looping their arms under her arms, around her chest, for balance and support. I could even get her up the stairs by walking with her, giving Dave a break from carrying her to bed every night. And now that Emily could speak, we started potty-training her (again). This time around was much quicker and within a few weeks she was out of diapers.

People kept saying the dreaded *I don't know how you do it.* Dave and I adjusted to this new life because we had no other choice. We had mourned our prior life and our fully functioning daughter when she was in the hospital and the first few months at home. Those tearful phone calls from the hospital, the tears that would creep up seemingly out of nowhere when we got home from the hospital, the loud swallows I would take when I heard her new voice, the frustration felt from changing a diaper on an eight-year-old ... those were the times I mourned the Emily I knew. We laid our prior life to rest.

The world kept spinning and that spring we joined it, but not with gusto. A new wheelchair-friendly baseball field was just built near our home, and I signed Emily up for a Miracle League baseball team. On Saturday mornings in the early summer, I drove Emily over to the field where she would play a ball game with other kids who had physical or cognitive disabilities. Each participant was assigned an aide who volunteered that Saturday—sometimes adults and sometimes baseball or softball players from local high schools. Emily sat in her wheelchair while the aide held the bat in her hand and swung at the pitch for her. She then pushed Emily around the bases. Some of the other players were able to get quality play time at the games, but it was hard for me to gauge if Emily really enjoyed it. All I knew was that I hated being there. Everyone in the stands clapped and cheered for Emily when the aide hit the ball for her. If only they could have seen her a year ago.

Emily's friends from school and the neighborhood wanted to visit with her. I warned the parents as much as I could that Emily was different now, but they were insistent. Vicki and her daughter were the first ones over to the house. Vicki kept telling me it was going to be all right when I told her I was worried her seven-year-old daughter would be upset. But really, it was I who held back my tears as I watched her friends, a reminder of her prior life, talk with Emily. I was the one who was uncomfortable, feeling the need to pick up the slack in the conversations between the kids. It was all without reason. Her friends were loving, compassionate and kind, and Emily truly enjoyed the visits, a smile on her face for each one. But I kept the visits short for everyone's sake. Emily fatigued quickly and most of her friends ran out of things to talk about, but mostly I didn't like the reminders of how much these kids were growing while mine was no longer keeping up with them.

Dave had heard from someone at work about a hiking trail that was wheelchair friendly less than an hour from our house. On a nice Saturday afternoon, shortly after learning of it, we decided to go on an adventure. We found the trail—a boardwalk—and started the mile-long trek with Emily comfortable in her wheelchair. We were all able to enjoy the breathtaking views of the majestic Rockies as Dave and I took turns wheeling her up the mountain, 9,000 feet above sea

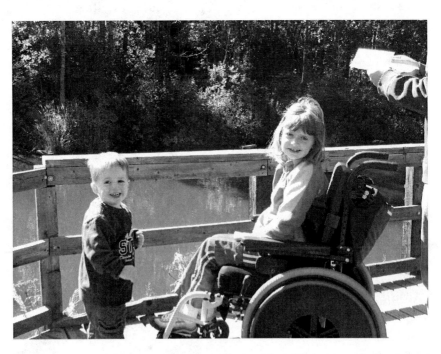

Ryan and Emily on our wheelchair accessible hike in the mountains of Colorado.

level. When we got to the top, we sat on a bench overlooking valleys filled with evergreens and aspens alongside snow-topped mountains and ate sandwiches we packed earlier that morning. Ryan found more rocks and sticks than he knew what to do with darting up and down the boardwalk and into the woods. The sunshine on my face and cool wind whipping my hair everywhere reminded me of how I felt when I first fell in love with Colorado. Being in the mountains still took my breath away. I was coming alive again.

I started taking more and more pride in Emily's progress instead of dwelling on what was lost. I could see, now, what tenacity she had waking up each day and getting through it with a smile and good cheer. She didn't ask, "Why me?" She didn't complain when she fell over. She just got up again. There was no frustration when somebody couldn't understand what she was saying. There was patience instead. There was never an "I'm too tired" when I forced her to walk to the car for her physical therapy session. She got up slowly, took each painstakingly slow step, all the way from the family room to the garage. And there was nothing but gratitude when her little brother, the one she had once held in her arms and fed a bottle to, was the one bringing her a toy because she couldn't get it herself. She was a graceful fighter.

⇒ 13 ⇐

School

Emily went back to school in the fall after her stroke, about one year later. She was still using her yellow wheelchair, but was now eating and drinking on her own, had had the G-tube removed, was out of diapers, and was speaking, albeit slowly. The aide that was hired to assist her two years before was eagerly awaiting her arrival that first day of third grade and Emily's IEP had been adjusted to accommodate her new needs. We anticipated fatigue being an issue as she hadn't been away from home in a stimulating environment for more than a few hours at a time and school was a long six hours. The week before school started, the staff created a quiet room. It was a closet converted to a beach, complete with a lounge chair and a view of waves painted on the walls. Here Emily could nap during the day if she needed to. Some teachers and staff at the school also had a custom toboggan made just for Emily. She would be able to go outside in the snow during recess with the other kids and be pulled around on this stunningly gorgeous sled that she comfortably fit in. The love we felt from the people surrounding us was immense and humbling. I never once faltered in leaving her for six hours a day in the hands of the staff at that school.

Emily was excited to go back to school, her confident nature undiminished. Her memory was still an issue, but it was hard to figure out as she still wasn't talking much and we filled in the empty air for her. On her first day back, Emily was greeted with more hugs and high-fives than were imaginable. I didn't know if we were just incredibly lucky to have the people we were surrounded by or if it was the fact that Emily herself was a happy, outgoing girl who was easy to be friends with, but seeing her in the circle of kids who had been in her life since preschool or kindergarten was now uplifting instead of heart-breaking. I had learned to stop seeing them as reminders of the past and to just be grateful that they were there for Emily.

Emily had joined a Brownie troop, part of the Girl Scouts organization, the spring before she had a stroke. One of the girls from her troop, Emma, who was also a classmate, asked Emily to come back to the troop and take part in the weekly meetings held at the school. At first, I laughed off this suggestion. It wasn't that Emily wouldn't enjoy the crafts that were done during the meetings or the friendships that came from sitting around a table with other little girls. I was the one who didn't want to sit at a table helping Emily with each task, after a long day of working and taking care of Ryan. But Emma was persistent, knowing her friend would enjoy the Brownie troop. So I took Emily to the next meeting after chugging a cup of coffee in the car on the way over. Emma was already there and ran out to greet us, holding the door open for me to push Emily through. Once I got Emily signed in, Emma asked, "Okay if I push her now?"

"Sure, Emma, just be careful."

Emma proceeded to push her all around the cafeteria, stopping to say hi to all the kids who were very chatty with Emily. Emily looked to be enjoying everything and got excited when they sat down to do a craft. And instead of me sitting next to Emily to help, Emma sat with her. The girls all around her helped Emily when she needed to cut a piece of paper or take the cap off the glue stick. I sat in the back of the room watching as Emily's every need was being tended to by friends. At the end of the meeting, after songs were sung, Emma expertly unlocked the wheelchair and safely delivered Emily back to me.

After that night, I realized that perhaps I had more of a problem with Emily's disability than Emily did. I made it a point for Emily to join in where she could. When we showed up at the next meeting, Emma greeted us again, but this time said, "Amy, I can help Emily if she needs it. It's fine for you not to stay."

I looked at Emily who smiled and said, "Emma can push me."

I trusted this nine-year-old little girl, so young and yet so knowing, because of her spirit. She never backed down from her friendship with Emily and was not shy to ask questions or get her needs met. And frankly, I was happy for the break. So, with that, I left Emily surrounded by her friends and of course let the troop leaders know that I was just a phone call away. We continued with that troop the rest of the season, leaving Emma in charge. There was never an issue, and Emma continued to be Emily's friend for years to come.

School continued to be an easy place for me to leave Emily for the day. It was, in all honesty, the only type of daycare available to us—allowing me to work and to have some time alone with Ryan. Her aide was with her, and the staff was more than accommodating. Emily, too, was still healing and growing, and we were seeing more and more of her functions returning. She talked more and more, the fatigue of the effort not nearly as debilitating. She was also taking more and more steps at home. The physical therapist ordered her a four-pronged cane to stabilize her as she walked. Although she spent most of her time at home in the beige reclining chair in the family room or sitting at the kitchen table, the cane gave her a sense of freedom. Emily could now get up by herself and walk to wherever she wanted to go without waiting for Dave or me to hold her hand.

Our life, though, still revolved around therapy appointments, exercises at home, and never-ending doctor appointments. She continued to have MRIs every three months to check the status of the tumors that still lingered in her brain. My anxiety regarding these MRIs remained the same. We felt like we were living with a time bomb; would this be the day it went off?

And we were also keeping up with an active almost-three-year-old. Ryan loved playing with trucks and superheroes, and our family room soon went from pink to a dark shade of blue. Cars, trucks, blocks and action figures littered the carpet. We would all spring into action, Ryan included, when we saw that Emily was on the move, clearing a wide path for her to walk. He would also bring Emily her toys to play with as well as say to her each night, "Time for pillows, Emmy!" This, we finally figured out, meant "It's time for your pills." Emily, by now, was taking about seven pills a night, and Ryan was well versed in the routine.

Both Dave and I were in our downstairs office one night after dinner and heard Emily ask, "Where's my cane?" I came out of the office and went to her, sitting in her chair in the family room, and looked around for the cane. I didn't see it.

"Emily, did you get up and go somewhere? Did you walk back without the cane?" I dumbly asked, confused.

"No," she replied, annoyed now. Of course she hadn't.

And then I heard a little giggle from the other room. I walked to the front of the house and there was Ryan, crouched in the corner of the formal living room, his hands over his mouth trying unsuccessfully to stifle his laughter, with the cane lying on the floor behind him. "Ryan!" I shouted. "You need to give that back to Emily." I had to stifle a giggle myself watching him run to Emily and hand her the cane. My laughter stopped after a few weeks of this "game," but bugging your sister is a normal, healthy thing. Sibling torture just looked a little different in our house.

That winter, when Emily was progressing ever so slowly but nicely, we got news that the tumor was growing again. I felt like there was no way, not with everything she had been through, that this could be possible. But even with my disbelief lingering in the air, the oncologist kept talking as if it was true. He stated that chemotherapy was not an option; we had exhausted the chemotherapies that worked for her type of tumor, and they were declared failures. Nothing new had come out in the few years since her last chemotherapy session. We agreed—surgery was no longer an option for Emily—so he referred us back to radiation oncology for a consult on radiation treatment.

Dave and I optimistically went to the consult. For every time that I thought *I wonder if this is it?* I had to tell myself to be positive. I couldn't live with the sadness that overwhelmed me every time I thought the worst. And although I knew that Dave grappled with the same thoughts—he must have—we didn't talk about it.

The doctor who met us said he reviewed Emily's case and had met with the oncologist. He recommended five days of radiation treatment. Just a short bit. He explained there were risks, but also reiterated that something needed to be done. What was left unsaid was that she might die from this tumor if left untreated.

Both Dave and I agreed that radiation seemed reasonable. Emily experienced no side effects from her first round of radiation and it was only five days of treatment this time. No hospital stays. No medicine rendering her fatigued and nauseous. Emily started the second round of radiation treatment two weeks later. At this point, going to the doctor to treat cancer felt as routine as dental cleanings.

The radiology clinic at the hospital was just as friendly and over-the-top welcoming as the first time around. Emily got through her five mornings there easily, and I was thankful to be able to go home and sleep in my own bed each night, not having to leave Ryan for a week. The treatment for this tumor re-growth was so fast and so limited in its side effects, Dave and I didn't have a chance to get out of denial that the tumor had grown again. Our life just continued. My family would keep asking how we were doing, and I would always respond, "Fine." And I was because I never fully bought into the fact that her cancer had returned yet again. Ah, denial, my best friend.

Shortly after that radiation stint, at the end of that winter, we decided to go on a beach vacation. Dave insisted that a change of scenery was necessary, at least for him. His adventurous spirit, always wanting to travel, never waned—even with our family limitations. Within a day of making the decision to go on vacation, we booked a one-bedroom condo on the Florida coast. The amount of work that went into that vacation—a nine-year-old in a wheelchair and a three-year-old little boy—was a bit daunting, but I kept my eye on the prize. It would be worth it to see the waves crashing on the sandy beach. And it was. It ended up being one of our best family vacations, perhaps because we probably needed it the most at that point in time.

⇛ 14 ⇚

Memory

Emily was back in school after missing a week for radiation and a few days for our beach vacation. The rest of her third grade year went by in a blur. Emily used her wheelchair all year and enjoyed the projects she worked on as well as the friendships she had. She was now known as the Thumb War champ and would gladly accept the Thumb War challenges from her fellow students (and even some parents). She was reading at grade level and doing math, although it proved to be her greatest struggle.

By the time Emily started fourth grade she was walking without the use of the cane. We realized her ability to walk independently in typical Emily fashion. She had been sitting in the beige chair in the family room watching *Lilo and Stitch* for the fortieth time when she walked to the entrance of the office, where Dave was sitting, and asked in her slow, thick speech, "Daddy, where's my cane?"

"What do you mean?" he asked. "How did you walk here without your cane?"

"I don't know."

Dave bolted out of his chair, surprised and worried that she would suddenly lose her balance, and they walked off looking for her cane. It was exactly where they thought it was—Ryan's hiding spot in the formal living room. They put the cane back in its typical spot next to Emily's chair, but Dave, laughing at the irony of her question, suggested to Emily that maybe she didn't need it anymore. From that point on, Emily didn't use her cane, and Ryan needed to find a new way to bug his big sister.

She was back to wearing an AFO on her right leg and walking around independently. I was back to dreading shoe shopping which typically resulted in tears (from me—not Emily). She was not running like before, but she could get around. Falling over became a weekly habit that would either frustrate her to the point of yelling or result in an "I'm okay!" depending on her mood. Her coordination had also improved to the point where she could play the Wii again. We had gotten a Wii video game console when it first came out years earlier, and Emily loved it. Finally, a game system where you only needed one hand to work the controller! She had finally recovered to a point where I wanted to burn the beige recliner in which Emily spent the last year sitting. Instead, I donated it and bought a new bright red chair to replace it.

Never having an easy path, as Emily was getting better and better neurologically, she started getting horribly bad stomachaches, waking up in the middle of the night screaming in pain. I would hear a scream at 2 a.m., rush to her room, tell her to stop screaming and then shut her windows. I didn't want the neighbors to think someone was getting murdered. My level of compassion, apparently, correlated to the hour of the day.

Within a week, Emily and I entered a new area of Children's Hospital for her to have an upper endoscopy and colonoscopy. Following this procedure, the doctor relayed that he found multiple ulcers in her stomach and intestines. "The ulcers are indicative of Crohn's disease. We'll wait for the biopsies to come back before making a definitive diagnosis, but that's what it looks like."

Sure enough, a few days later we got the call confirming the biopsies were consistent with Crohn's disease, giving Emily yet another medical issue to live with. Crohn's disease, we learned, can cause abdominal pain and problems with bowel movements. Emily already had bowel issues as a side effect of her chemotherapy treatment, and those issues never actually resolved. Her oncologist told me after Emily's colonoscopy that studies had just come out linking some chemotherapy medicines to Crohn's disease, which was likely why Emily now had it. The good news was that there were medicines to alleviate the symptoms of the disease. The bad news was this was a lifelong disease with no cure. It would just need be managed, and she most likely would have "flares" every now and then.

Medicines to manage Crohn's disease were added to Emily's pill box. The nurse at Emily's school was updated with the latest diagnosis and treatment plan. Dave and I took this news as just one more thing. More of an annoyance for her and us. One more thing to manage on our end and one more thing for her to endure. The medicine she was on compromised her immune system, not as severely as chemotherapy, but it left Emily a bit more susceptible to colds and infections. On the upside, she was still on a low-dose antibiotic to manage the chronic UTIs from her refluxing kidney. I felt they balanced each other out as we didn't really notice any increase in the number of colds Emily suffered from. Emily's middle-of-the-night stomachaches went away, and now a GI specialist was added to the list of doctors we saw routinely every three months.

It was also during fourth grade that the school aide started relaying feedback about Emily's progress in school. She was having a difficult time with the work and the aide had to help her more and more. For instance, Emily did not have trouble reading the words of a story, but often she didn't remember what she just read. And any lesson beyond simple addition and subtraction was lost on Emily. After a meeting with her teachers, we realized that Emily's memory was failing her. Learning new things was incredibly difficult. It wasn't that she had lost cognitive functioning; it was that she couldn't seem to learn more due to her short-term memory deficit. We started to worry at this point that perhaps the radiation treatment was also contributing to her memory loss.

We realized then that this was why Emily no longer wanted to watch new movies or new TV shows. She was only interested in programs that she had already seen when she was younger. She knew the storylines. She knew the characters. It was difficult to be interested in a movie when you couldn't remember the first 20 minutes or keep track of the characters. This was also why she had no interest in new books, even though she had no problem reading the words in them. And now we understood when she complained that school was hard.

Her teachers tried applying tactics that would help Emily function without her memory. Lists were made, charts were hung on the wall, and calendars were created. All these tricks worked to a degree. The problem was that she needed reminders to use them daily for months or even years before she would remember to use them herself.

In addition to memory problems, she was slower. Everything

was slow—her walking, her talking, and her reactions. Prior to the stroke, Emily's favorite class was art, so I was surprised when Emily's aide told me she was getting very frustrated in her art class. By the end of the year, Emily would practically be in tears, and the aide would often take her to the quiet beach room instead of art. It turned out that Emily just couldn't keep up with the other kids in class. They would be asked to paint a picture, and Emily would only be halfway done before they went on to the next project which frustrated her. The same thing happened in music class. All Emily had to do in this class was sing along with the chorus, but it, too, moved too fast. She couldn't read the words to the song in time with the pace of the song. They aide said she did not participate, just moved her lips. Listening to the aide tell me these things was difficult, but since I wasn't the one witnessing them, I could shove those comments to the side.

Beyond the difficulties with academics, I finally figured out that she couldn't tell me about her day. She compensated by being vague. I would ask, "Who did you sit with at lunch today?" And she would respond, "The same friends as always." "What was your favorite part of school today?" "Seeing my friends." It took us a while to figure out that she knew the right answers and never really gave details, just enough fluff to answer the questions to my satisfaction. If someone said hello to her in a hallway, she would smile, wave and say hello. I'd ask her who that person was, and she would shrug and say, "I don't know."

This also meant that any time she wasn't with me, I was dependent on who was in charge to let me know what happened during that time. I couldn't depend on Emily to let me know that she was hurt, in danger, or even really enjoyed something while out of my sight or reach. Leaving Emily meant entrusting her to the people surrounding her—a scary thing to wrap my head around.

The upside to her memory loss, Dave and I both realized, was that when we lost our cool, which happened more often than not, Emily forgot. She asked one weekend, repeatedly, "When are we going to Nana and Grandpa's house?" We had talked for a few days about going to their house to swim with her cousins, and she was really looking forward to it.

After the sixth time asking within a 20-minute period, I

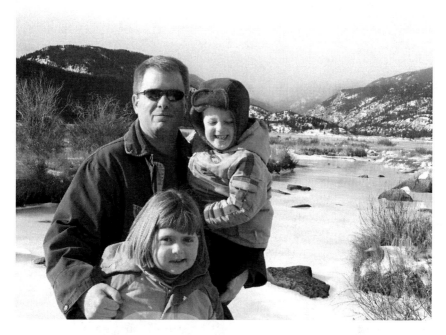

Dave, holding Ryan, and Emily on a trip to the mountains.

responded with furrowed brows and arms in the air, "Emily! For the last time, we are going after we eat lunch!"

She put her head down and whimpered, "I'm sorry."

I immediately felt miserable. She never intended to be annoying with her persistent questions. She also hated to displease anyone.

I got down to her level and looked in her eyes and apologized. "No, I'm sorry. You asked several times—I lost my patience."

She said, "It's okay."

Five minutes later she asked when we were going to Nana and Grandpa's house. All was forgotten.

≋ 15 ≋

Summertime Blues

The summer before Emily started fifth grade was rough. Ryan had just completed a year of preschool and was easy to entertain. Emily, however, was dependent on routine. Routine, in fact, became our best friend. Emily could count on routine and not rely on her memory to understand what came next in our day. That summer I would get the Play-Doh out and after four minutes she had lost interest and wanted to play kitchen instead. After 20 minutes of playing kitchen she wanted to watch a TV show. Things that kept her attention were drawing pictures and writing stories, so we stocked up on markers, paper, pens and notebooks and counted our blessings when she would sit for more than 45 minutes working on a picture.

It seemed that because of her memory impairment, Emily was stuck at seven years old while her friends were well into their pre-teen years. This made it difficult for Dave and me to get together with our friends who had a child the same age as Emily. Before, the kids would play together while the parents visited—an enjoyable time for all. But now, Emily wanted to play dolls or draw pictures while the other girls wanted to talk about boys or play on their handheld devices. And although none of the kids balked or resisted playing with Emily, it felt forced and made me uncomfortable. Thankfully, she had cousins, aunts, uncles and grandparents who doted on her and were most of her social engagement outside of school.

I didn't know of any camps for kids with special needs, and I certainly could not sign her up for the regular camps and classes held in our town. Instead, in between finding a few hours here and there to work, I became her playmate, camp leader, chef, personal assistant, driver, physical trainer and overall cruise director. Ryan, and sometimes his friends, also played with Emily that summer. The boys loved to play with Emily's toy kitchen and they all played "house" together, including Emily in the game.

Our friends who lived next door had moved away, and a family with three young boys moved in—resulting in instant friendships for Ryan. We spent much of that summer sitting on lawn chairs on our driveway. The mom of the boys from next door, Alicia, would join us and the three of us would chit chat while boys zoomed around us on scooters and bikes. Emily would often sit with her notebook on her lap while Alicia and I gave her story ideas or requests for pictures which she happily drew for us.

Somehow, we got through the summer. Every time I felt I reached my breaking point, which was often, we got through another day. I counted down the days until Emily went back to school. She needed that routine, and I needed her to be busy without me. Her memory problems resulted in countless, monotonous questions and conversations every day. *SpongeBob, Lilo and Stitch*, and *Cinderella* played on a loop all summer long in my family room. I would hope for those rare times that a TV show or a movie would hold her interest to give me more than a few minutes of freedom. She still went to bed by 8 p.m., though, which was my saving grace. We didn't go out much, not many people stopped over anymore, and there were only reruns on TV. But I had two hours of uninterrupted time to myself every night between Emily's bedtime and when I collapsed in my bed. Those two hours restored my sanity that seemed to diminish as the day, and year, went on.

Finally, the end of August arrived, signaling the start of the school year. Emily went back to her school for fifth grade, and Ryan started his second year of preschool. I was, again, giddy to drop both off. And both were just as excited as I was to go back to school.

Within weeks of the school year starting, though, I received a phone call from Emily's principal. She wanted to talk to me about a classroom at a nearby elementary school that she thought Emily would thrive in. I was confused because Emily enjoyed her current school, had an aide who helped her, and seemed to have lots of friends who played with Emily during recess. But I didn't argue and agreed to, at least, visit the class with Emily and her aide the next day.

We walked into the classroom of the other elementary school, a few blocks further than our neighborhood school, and I immediately thought, *Nope. Not the right place for Emily.* Although the classroom was large and decorated festively, there were kids who were outspoken and loud, some who flapped their hands, some who talked differently, and one who didn't talk at all. *Why on earth am I here?*

The teacher greeted us warmly and talked with Emily like they were old friends. "It's so good to see you, Emily!"

Emily smiled, "It's nice to see you too."

"I'd love to introduce you to my friends...." The teacher went on talking directly to Emily as she introduced her personally to the other 10 students in the classroom. She then directed Emily to a desk she had prepared for Emily's visit that day.

Emily sat at the open desk and started talking with a girl her age sitting at the desk next to her. They laughed together and were comparing outfits, complimenting each other on their sparkly shirts. The teacher then started a lesson and included Emily, who answered a question and watched as other kids participated too. The teacher went at her speed, pausing long enough for the students to take in what was just said as well as to form their answers, giving them an opportunity to participate. I looked over at her aide, sitting across the room, and noticed tears running down her face. When we left that afternoon, the aide, tears still streaming down her face, said, "Finally, a place where Emily can be comfortable. This is exactly what she needs."

This aide, who had been by Emily's side for three years now, knew the struggles Emily was having in school much more intimately than I did. I could shrug off the fact that Em got frustrated with art or music or math. Her aide actually dealt with the frustration day in and day out. "How amazing," the aide continued, "it would be for Emily not to always feel left behind or that she's not smart enough." Hearing those words helped me clearly see the Emily of the present, not the past. Not only did Emily fit in here, she belonged here. She could learn and thrive in this setting, and maybe even make a friend who enjoyed the same games and toys that she enjoyed.

"That was so fun!" Emily said when we got in the car.

"What do you think about going to school here?" I asked with my new perspective.

"Yes!"

At home I described our experience to Dave. He thought it sounded wonderful, especially all the things they would be doing, like cooking in the kitchen attached to the classroom. At the end of the week Emily had a good-bye pizza party at her elementary school. There were a lot of tears shed that day at the school that had looked out for Emily's best interests every day she was there, from providing an aide to knowing when they could no longer provide the best environment for her.

I drove Emily to her new school the following Monday and left her in a classroom knowing she was in good hands. After all, she and her aide were a package deal. Her aide agreed to go to the new school with her. Emily thrived in this new environment and no longer complained about going to school.

Emily had made friends in her new class and enjoyed a play date here or there, but I soon learned that play dates with other kids who had special needs required a lot of work. Emily had always played with typically developing kids who could do things like take caps off markers, decide on a game to play, and keep the conversation going. When Emily was with a friend who also needed help, it meant that either me or the other parent had to do the helping, talking, and decision making. It just took a lot more coordination and effort on the parents' part and sometimes, honestly, it wasn't quite worth the effort.

In the spring of that year I started to panic. Not about Emily's health or our long-term future. I just positively dreaded the long summer fast approaching between Emily's fifth and sixth grades and before Ryan started kindergarten. I couldn't fathom another summer of *SpongeBob*, drawing, and playing kitchen. I frantically looked through every camp brochure searching for something that might be a fit for Emily but came up short. I couldn't find any activity to sign her up for.

Sure enough, summer break started as promised, and the questions, the monotonous conversations, *SpongeBob*, and the drawings took over. We decided to break up the summer with a trip to the mountains over the Fourth of July which proved to be a fantastic idea. The break from the heat, along with the mountain scenery, put everyone in a good mood. The balcony of our condo overlooked a lake where fireworks were set off on the Fourth. For the first time, the four of us sat outside and watched the fireworks together. We didn't have crowds to navigate or a late bedtime to contend with, making the usual Fourth of July events a no-go. We woke Emily up at 9 after she fell asleep on the couch two hours earlier to watch the spectacle. We finally did, as a family, something the rest of the nation did year after year. The night felt magical.

Back at home, we worked hard trying to figure out things to do together as a family. Doing something physical was out of the question, even though Ryan would have appreciated it. We lived near some of the best ski resorts in the country and couldn't take advantage of them as a family. Although I felt bad that we were not exposing Ryan to the sport, I was fine not skiing. I was horrible at it and it was expensive. Dave missed it but didn't complain about the days not spent on the slopes. Hiking was my thing—it was easy, there were usually breathtaking views, there was wildlife to see, and it was cheap. But we certainly couldn't do that with Emily. One thing we found that we all enjoyed was "Jeeping." We could sit the kids in the back of Dave's Jeep and go four-wheeling through the mountains.

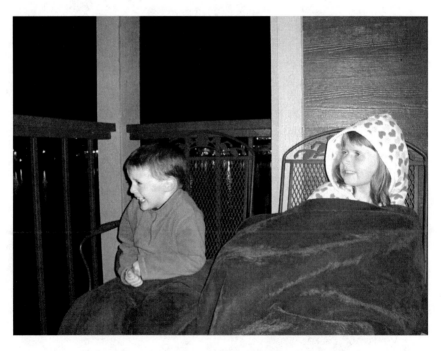

Ryan and Emily watching the 4th of July fireworks.

Usually we stopped near the top of a trail for a picnic lunch and let Ryan run through the woods while either Dave or myself sat with Emily on the picnic blanket.

Later that summer, in another fit of boredom, we got a dog—a West Highland Terrier we named Lucy, pronounced with a Cuban accent. She fit right into our household, and I had something new to distract me from the mundaneness of our routine. Lucy loved to nap next to Emily and chase Ryan through the yard. Most of all, she loved chewing on Ryan's toys. Ryan eventually got over his loss and concluded that Captain America was still a hero even though he was missing a leg and Batman could fly with a shredded cape. It didn't take long for me to have more pictures of the dog than I did of the kids. Before we knew it, summer ended, and we had survived.

Ryan was officially toting a big backpack to take to his first day of "real" school. He started kindergarten in Emily's old classroom with the same teacher while Emily entered sixth grade at the wonderful school she started last year. Ryan was just as confident as Emily going into class that first day. After all, he'd been watching Emily go to school all his life and was ready for it to be his turn. By now, he was soft spoken, smart, and still interested in anything related to superheroes. He made friends easily and became best buds with a boy in his class who happened to be the little brother of one of Emily's old classmates. I was able to see and keep up with all the parents of Emily's original friends as they dropped their now–sixth graders off at that same school. Although I no longer felt the sting, the reminder that their kids had moved on, were growing like they were supposed to, I felt like an outsider.

Emily's health stabilized, if you could call it that. Her every-three-month MRIs turned into every-six-month MRIs because the tumor was proving to be stable. This was excellent if not scary news as we now had to endure a full six months before sighing in relief that the tumor hadn't grown. However, we now had appointments with the GI doctor almost monthly. Emily's management of her Crohn's was much like epilepsy. The doctor changed medication or dose with every flare-up or setback Emily experienced. It became hard to believe that some of medicine wasn't just guesswork.

We felt more tied to home than before between Emily's unpredictable seizure activity and the abdominal pain, along with hours spent in the bathroom. If we did an activity with Emily, we needed it to be short and quick. It got to the point where we dreaded the weekends, no longer feeling able to even enjoy a Jeep ride through the mountains.

Our dismal moods that year were also fueled by the fact that Dave and I were coming to terms with Emily's prognosis. She had a severe cognitive disability that was proving to be permanent. We struggled to cope with now knowing she would never grow up and go to college. She wouldn't marry or have kids. And she would live with us forever. It wasn't an overnight revelation; these thoughts crept in and out of our minds over several months and years until we accepted it. Even once we seemed to have accepted these thoughts as truth, there were still times that we fought against it. There were uncalled-for outbursts at each other or anyone who passed by us in a moment of unseen grief. We talked with each other about these feelings, but not often. We didn't know *how* to talk about these things, topics that seemed taboo. We certainly didn't talk with our friends and family about these revelations. I felt we were the only ones going through it and that people just didn't understand our reality. I felt more alone than ever before.

Dave was also growing restless with his job. He watched as his colleagues moved on to bigger assignments while he maintained his three-day work week assignment in order to help at home. Elisa, knowing he was frustrated at work, let him know of a remote opportunity that was in his field. He quickly applied for that job and was offered the position, but it took a long time to decide if he should go forward with the change of jobs. After several long conversations, going back and forth about leaving a position he'd been at for more than 15 years, he finally accepted the remote position.

The new job energized Dave and gave him something different to focus on although he found it was lonely working remotely. Now he really had no other adults to interact with throughout the week— just me. But he was happy with the job itself, and it was nice for me to have someone home all day to keep me company. My job had also grown mundane, even mind-numbing, certainly not the stimulation it had once given me. But I couldn't argue with my part-time hours and remote status. Ease, when I could get it, trumped everything else.

That winter, at what seemed the height of our lonely despair, heartache hit us in yet another way. It was a typical school morning—the kids were finishing breakfast and watching cartoons as I let Lucy out for her morning business. I stood in the bay window in the kitchen with my cup of coffee while the dog was out, watching her hop through the eight inches of snow covering our yard, and then proceeded to pack lunches for Ryan and Emily. Once the lunches were made, I opened the back door and called for her. I heard and saw nothing. Sighing out of frustration, I yelled loudly now, "Lucy!" Still nothing. Aggravated, I threw snow boots on over my pajama bottoms to trudge through the snow and find the dog. I did a quick look through the back yard but couldn't find her. A pit formed in my stomach as I looked at the time, realizing I needed to get the kids to school. I ran upstairs, got myself and both kids dressed, then sent the kids back downstairs. I shook Dave awake and told him I couldn't find the dog—he'd need to go look for her while I took the kids to school.

Without saying anything to the kids about the missing dog, I drove them to school. I quickly rushed home to find Dave in the kitchen waiting for me.

"Did you find her?"

"Yes, but not alive. Coyotes got her," Dave said quickly.

"*No!*" I burst into tears. "How do you know?" This couldn't be true.

"I found part of her body. And there are track marks all through the yard. You can see where they hopped the fence and grabbed her." He rattled this off too fast for me to grasp, even though we'd been hearing the coyotes all winter long, their yip-yip-yipppeee calls waking us most nights.

"Oh my God." *My poor Lucy.* The sobs came quickly and didn't end for roughly three days. Dave held me until he needed to leave for a lunch with colleagues who were in town. I then stood at the kitchen window, crying on the phone with my mother, and watched as a coyote stood just outside our split-rail fence which was covered with chicken wire, and stared at me.

"Get out of here!" I yelled through the glass, deafening my mother still on the phone. Of course, he didn't hear me and continued to sit, licking his paw.

"I hate this godforsaken state," I told my mother.

I spent the remainder of the day useless, just crying. I made it to Emily's school at three o'clock to pick her up. I didn't say anything, wanting to wait until we were home. From there, we went to Ryan's school to pick him up. The teacher opened the door and all the kids filed out into the field. While Ryan was playing with friends, I pulled the teacher aside and let her know what had happened. She gave me a hug and said she'd keep an eye on Ryan.

At home, we all sat on the couch and I broke the news to the kids. I started crying all over again. Ryan was quick to join me, resulting in Dave getting misty-eyed. I cried now for the heartache felt by Ryan losing his first "real" pet. Emily was quiet. She didn't cry, just repeated, "It's very sad." She then asked if she could draw a picture. As I got out her drawing supplies and sat her at the counter, I prayed that she would remember that Lucy was gone. I couldn't handle her asking repeatedly where the dog was.

Ryan and I spent the rest of the day crying, and every time Emily looked at us, she would say, "It's very sad."

"Yes," I would tell her. At least our constant tears were reminding Emily that we lost Lucy.

Elisa called me the next day to see how I was doing. In between my sobs, she said, "I've never seen you this upset before. And you've gone through some pretty horrific stuff with Emily."

"Emily never died!" I shouted. And maybe that was it. Maybe it was that Lucy had died and Emily had come close and I was blurring the lines. Or maybe it was just the straw that broke the camel's back. This had come after several months of waning, not feeling like we were experiencing life anymore, and this just solidified it. Perhaps my three days of tears were shed for not only mourning our dog but mourning our life as well.

Ten days after Lucy died, Dave told us to get in the car without telling us where we were going. Only after we were on the road for five minutes did he say that we were getting another dog.

"Seriously?!" I didn't know what to think of this idea.

"Yes," he replied. "I can't take the sadness in our house anymore."

And that was how Sandy, a Soft-Coated Wheaten Terrier, who would grow to be 40 pounds, joined our family. She was a furry blob of a dog that had no body awareness and would flop on the couch next to you, half on your lap, half falling off the couch. And we loved this silly girl. Dave was right. It was a good cure for the sadness that hung in the air that winter.

I called the Colorado Department of Wildlife to ask what we could do about the coyotes near our house, considering we had a puppy. They told me I could shoot them if they were on our property. I laughed, thinking how that would look in my suburban neighborhood. As much as I wanted them gone, that was not going to happen. "What else?" I asked, looking for a more reasonable solution.

"You can throw rocks at them and yell; that should scare them away." Although that still sounded unreasonable, I was no Annie Oakley and I needed the coyotes gone.

I had Ryan help me gather a bunch of rocks and filled the pockets of my winter coat. I put on my coat, armed, ready to take Sandy out every few hours. On more than one occasion, I threw a rock at a coyote and yelled at it to go away. Each time I threw a rock, the coyote ran in the other direction. It worked.

The weather was getting nicer, which meant the coyotes were less of a threat. It also meant more outside time for Ryan. One afternoon, sitting with Alicia and Emily as the boys showed off their light saber tricks on our driveway, I learned that Alicia had several runners in her family but she admitted that running was not her thing. We were able to agree on this. "Running is not my thing, either. I ran a 10K once, but I'm really not a runner," I told her.

"Really? That's a long race for someone who doesn't run."

"Ha, I almost died! Actually, though, I've been toying with the idea of running again. Dave's sister wants to do a marathon, and she asked me to run it with her. She has one of those 'couch to marathon' training guides that she sent to me," I admitted to Alicia. I needed to do something to get out of my funk. I wanted a goal, something to look forward to. Maybe this time I would even feel that "runner's high" and get skinny.

Alicia pondered for a moment before asking, "Can I see that training guide? I have zero interest in running a marathon, but maybe we can do a few training runs together?"

That Saturday, Alicia and I agreed to run one mile. At the end of that mile we high-fived each other, beaming at the fact that we ran the entire mile and didn't collapse. We confidently made plans to run again. We would drop the kids off at school and go for a run, following our guide. Typically, this meant that we ran two or three times during the week and did a longer run on Saturdays.

I still hated running. But I loved the time with Alicia and the fresh air. I loved that I had only a grown up to talk with, and there was absolutely nothing else to think about—other than breathing. Dave was fine with my running but started getting irritated once our Saturday runs reached seven or eight miles. It took me a long time to run that distance and by the time I came home I was exhausted. He was stuck at home watching the kids all morning by himself and was ready to do something fun when I got home, and all I wanted to do was lie on the couch. Really, all I *could* do was lie on the couch. My body was not recovering easily from those long runs.

I kept running even though Dave was growing lonely and tired with this routine. I was committed to doing that marathon with his sister, Tammy. But by now, I was also battling knee pain and my recovery time was lasting into Sundays. In the midst of spending nearly all my spare time running, Dave suggested we take a cruise with the kids. He needed something to look forward to. I wasn't sure how the logistics of staying in a tiny room with a tinier bathroom would work for our family, but I was in no position to say no to Dave who had been sacrificing so much for me these days. Thankfully, he had the same concerns and went ahead and booked two adjoining rooms (we ate Ramen for dinner for several weeks to pay for this, but travel was a priority for Dave).

A month later we flew to New Orleans and boarded a boat headed to Mexico, Honduras, and Belize. Emily and Ryan were good travelers, practiced with all the trips we had done back to the East Coast from Colorado. This trip proved to be no different. Getting two rooms was the key to our happiness. We had rooms with balconies, though, which worried me, so I barricaded the doors to the balcony with the heavy desk chair so that neither Ryan nor Emily would be tempted to go on the balcony without me or Dave. We also slept with the door between our rooms open.

The first night of the cruise, I heard Emily call my name in the middle of the night. I went to her bedside, and she just wanted to know what time it was—a usual question for her, wanting to know if the magical 5 appeared on the clock allowing her to wake for the day.

The second night I faintly heard "Mom." At first, I thought I dreamt it because it was so faint, but then I heard it again. I went to the kids' room, and panic seized me when I saw Emily wasn't in her bed. Ryan was sound asleep in his bed. I looked in the bathroom. Empty. I heard the faint "Mom" again, from the *outside hallway*. I whipped open the door to the cabin and there stood Emily. All she said was, "There you are. Is it time to get up yet?"

I ushered her back in the room and examined the door handle. I'm not sure how she was able to figure out the lock and swing the door open. After that, I barricaded that door as well. Other than that incident, it was a mostly stress-free vacation. When we stopped in Roatán, Honduras, we splurged and hired a cab driver for the day. He brought us through town where Ryan and Emily got see local kids getting dismissed from school for lunch, running home. He then brought us to the most quiet, beautiful beach we had ever seen.

While sitting on the beach, Dave turned to me and asked, "Where's Ryan?"

I looked at him lazily, drifting in and out of a nap on a makeshift beach towel made of my sweatshirt, sitting next to Emily. "What?"

"Where'd Ryan go?"

He wasn't in a panic, the serenity of the beach overtaking Dave as well. We looked up and down the beach and couldn't see him. But then, straight ahead of us, in the *ocean*, was our five-year-old son happily swimming by himself. That was enough to wake us out of our beach stupor.

The rest of the trip was amazing. Although we didn't enjoy any of the evening entertainment on the ship, Dave and I sat on our balcony and gazed at the stars every night while the kids were in bed. I even continued my marathon training. The cruise ship had a track on the top floor of the boat which I used almost daily for short runs.

Back home, Alicia and I were up to 15 miles on our Saturday runs. Once we reached that point, we decided to do a local half-marathon that was coming up in a few weeks. That was the most Alicia said she wanted to do, sticking to her guns about no marathons. Two weeks later Alicia and I crossed the finish line of that half-marathon. We ran the entire race, not stopping to walk once, although our time on that race might cause one to question that claim. I was proud we accomplished the 13.1 mile run which made it hard not to have Dave, Emily and Ryan there to greet me at the finish line. It was too difficult to figure out the logistics of parking and getting Emily through that crowd, especially not knowing what time I was going to finish. So I quickly said goodbye to Alicia, celebrating with her family, and drove home to let Dave and the kids know that I did it. I cried the entire way home, feeling sorry for myself and angry at our situation. I couldn't even have my husband and kids at the finish line.

I decided after that race that there was no way I was going to run a marathon. The half-marathon took it out of me, and my knees never forgave me. It was also too hard to get that training time in. I was useless on the weekends—gone for the entire morning on a long run and then unable to function fully the rest of the day, continuing into Sunday. It wasn't fair to Dave or the kids. I called Tammy and broke the news to her. She understood, of course, and I told her that either Dave or I would be there at the finish line for her. I might have abandoned her on the run, but she would have someone at the finish line. That, I learned, was important.

16

Sky High Hope

Emily was wrapping up her sixth grade at the new school, which meant that she would need to move on to a junior high school for the next few years. To say I was sad to leave this classroom, the same one I was reluctant to have Emily join initially, would be an understatement. Emily was able to learn things in this class that I didn't think was possible given her memory deficiencies.

The end of the school year also signaled the start of the dreaded summer. God, I hated summer break. We didn't have anything planned for this break, having just taken a pricey cruise. The anxiety of not knowing, or rather *knowing*, how we were going to fill those long summer days was starting to set in. But then my friend Vicki called and asked if she could stop by after work. She started a new job that was associated with a camp for kids with chronic illnesses and wanted to tell me about it.

"They do arts and crafts, archery, fishing, boating, and horse-back riding!" Vicki told me, excited to share this with me in hopes that Emily would go.

"It sounds great, but could Emily participate?"

"Yes, it's specifically for kids who have special needs. Doctors and nurses are the ones running the camp—they take the week off and volunteer there. She'd be in great hands."

"Where is it?"

"At a horse ranch in the mountains, a few hours from here."

"A few hours from here? Wait, is this a sleepaway camp?!"

"Yup. And Emily would love it," Vicki said, knowing Emily's confident nature.

"I don't think so," I quickly responded. How on earth could

Emily stay at a camp for a week, in the mountains, with all of her needs?

"They are totally equipped to handle Emily, and Emily would love it," she said again.

She left me with the literature to review and the paperwork to fill out if I decided to sign her up for the week in June the camp was being offered. The next morning, I called the woman who headed up this camp each year, and she repeated what Vicki told me: "Emily would love it and, yes, we can handle her."

After talking more about it with Dave, we agreed to sign Emily up for the camp. However, we both thought it a good idea to book a hotel room 20 minutes from the campsite for the week she was there in case anything happened. Emily was thrilled at the idea of going away to camp—she would have friends to play with all week long. Plus, she could ride horses, which she loved, thanks to her cousin, Katie.

The day finally came for us to deliver Emily to camp. I had stuffed a suitcase full of any items she might need during a one-month long excursion to both the North Pole and Amazon jungle. I wrote down paragraphs explaining her medications, diagnoses, physical limitations and bowel habits. I packed her pill bottles in the Ziploc freezer bag like the paperwork told me to do. We were ready. We arrived at the check-in right on time, after climbing a road that required 4-wheel drive it was so rocky and steep. The terrain was *not* conducive to someone with a right-side weakness who had trouble with balance. Yet here I was, handing my daughter off to strangers.

After an hour of welcoming Emily, introducing us to all the staff, and showing us her cabin, the director told Dave and me to leave. She literally told us, as we were sitting in her cabin, "Okay, you really need to leave now."

And we just sat there staring at her.

"Emily, can you say good-bye to your parents?"

"See ya later, alligator!" Emily said.

We finally got up and kissed Emily good-bye. As we walked to the car, I turned around—I forgot to mention that Emily's an early riser. And I never checked to see if the toilet paper was on the left-hand side. I turned to Dave, "I didn't tell them how early she wakes up. And the toilet paper—did you see if it's on the left side for her?"

"I didn't notice." He paused, looking around. "Maybe we should go, though. You can call the director when we get to the hotel."

It was a bizarre, unreal feeling to leave Emily with strangers. As soon as we got to the hotel, I called the director and left a message. I didn't relax until I heard back from her that evening. She reported that Emily had actively participated in all the games they played that afternoon, ate a good dinner, sang songs around the fire, and quickly fell asleep back in the cabin with her cabinmates. She ended the conversation saying, "How about I call you if there's an issue? Otherwise, let's just assume she's having a great time." In other words, relax.

Feeling more comfortable, Dave, Ryan and I explored our mountain resort. We packed Ryan's scooter and let him ride it all over the windy, hilly roads. We had dinner together, just the three of us, and went on a hike. It felt quite freeing exploring the area with our son who didn't have any limitations. But we soon realized on the hike that Emily couldn't take all the blame for us missing out on these marvelous walks through the woods. Hiking with a six-year-old meant stopping every few minutes and listening to whining all the other minutes. It took us two hours to hike less than a few miles.

After four days at the mountain resort, we headed home. Dave had to get back to work, and we were confident that Emily was doing well, having not heard any more from the camp. A few days later, I drove my parents and Ryan back up to the rocky camp in the mountains to pick up Emily. I was beside myself with excitement to see her after this big adventure. As we walked to the point where parents were supposed to meet the campers, Emily walked by, holding hands with a young counselor, and they were laughing about something. "Emily! Hi! Em!" I was waving and shouting like a crazy woman.

She turned to me, smiled and waved, but then kept walking away and laughing with this girl. *What the hell?* My mom just looked at me and shook her head. "C'mon, Mother Lion, let's go to the waiting area."

It turned out that Emily had an amazing time. We watched a

slideshow of the week, put together by the camp directors, and Emily was in lots of pictures either smiling or laughing. She played games, sang camp songs, did archery, fished, and rode horses. In fact, the family that donated their ranch land to this camp to use every summer "gave" Emily a horse. They selected Emily because of her great attitude and spirit, they said. Emily got to name this horse (Bruno), helped change his shoes, groomed him, and rode him daily. Once I found out about this gift, I asked the incredibly generous ranch owner, "You keep Bruno here, right?" He laughed and said, "Of course!" But he made sure to tell us that anytime Emily wanted to ride Bruno, we could just drive on over. The kindness and love toward Emily and our family never went unfelt or unappreciated.

The overnight camp, and our overnight stay in the mountains, got us through the first month of summer break with barely a headache. The excitement and planning leading up to it, the week away, and the pictures and notes to look through for weeks after kept us all entertained. But then reality slowly crept back.

The days became long and monotonous again. Work was boring,

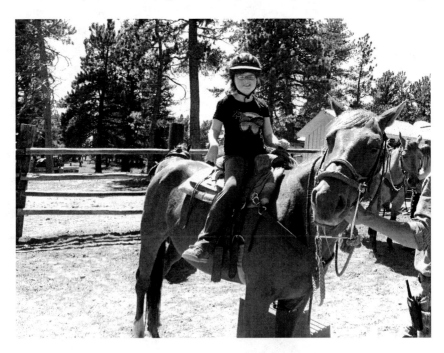

Emily riding "her" horse Bruno.

and entertaining Emily was a struggle. Dave, although happy with his work, was bored otherwise. Ryan seemed to be the only one with a wide circle of friends and things going on. He had numerous play-dates and events at pools and parks all summer long. It was hard to talk with the moms at these events because I had Emily to occupy and keep safe instead of chitchatting. Many times, I just dropped Ryan off as either the environment wasn't conducive to Emily or she wasn't feeling well.

The Fourth of July came and went, and I was wishing for the celebration we had the previous year. Instead, Dave, Ryan and I watched fireworks being shot off in distant towns from our deck, Emily sleeping in her bed upstairs. The following week, though, I had something to look forward to: I had a job interview for a completely remote position with a large company. It was for more hours than I was currently working, but I was desperate for a change and welcomed a challenge.

Three weeks later I was offered the position and accepted it with little thought. I didn't tell the person who offered me the job about my home life, since this was a completely remote position. However, I learned that I would need to attend a one-week training in Southern California once I started the job at the end of August. Dave was fine with this and encouraged the change, as he knew how desperate I was feeling with my current job status. With him working from home, handling the kids while I was away was manageable.

Emily was scheduled for a routine MRI the week before I started the new job and was to fly to Los Angeles. It didn't occur to me that we would hear anything but "the tumor is stable" at this visit. I should have known better.

I looked at the MRI films with the doctor explaining the growth, which I could see myself. I looked at him with desperation. *No more,* I thought in my head. The doctor apologized. He said he would need some time and would meet with other doctors before giving me a direction for treatment options. I dumbly explained that I was starting a new job next week and that I was supposed to be in California for the week.

"Will you have your cell phone with you, or do you want me to call Dave?" he asked.

"Yes, can you call me after you get a plan? The training is

informal—I can take the call." Thankfully, I was just meeting with the person who was previously in this role. We were meeting at my hotel and coffee shops for her to get me up to speed over the course of the week.

At home that afternoon, I broke the news to Dave. The scary thing about hearing your daughter's cancer has come back not once, not twice, but five times, is that it becomes very matter of fact. But this time, I decided that I didn't want her to have any more treatment. I had thought about it since her Crohn's diagnosis and since the last round of radiation. The treatments were no longer worth the damage they were causing her body. I didn't verbalize my feelings to Dave, though. I wanted to hear what the doctor had to say about treatment options first. Plus, I assumed Dave felt the same way as I did, so there was no need to say the words out loud.

Dave was numb like I was. This was no news to us anymore. I hated that I had to leave the next week. But I had already quit my old job, and there wasn't another choice. That Monday, I flew to L.A. and stayed in Calabasas, just outside of Malibu. It was a gorgeous area that was lost on me. I was miserable. I wanted to be near Emily, Dave, and Ryan.

It was a terrible time to be left alone in a hotel room with only my thoughts to keep me company. I couldn't stop picturing Emily's death. I prayed she wouldn't feel pain or be scared. I planned her funeral. I worried for Ryan, how he would handle losing a sister. I wondered if he would remember her. I cried. How could you not when you're planning your twelve-year-old daughter's funeral? Only when daylight came and my colleague appeared at my door for our meeting did I put those thoughts away. How easy it became to compartmentalize the thoughts in my head with all the practice I've had. It was time to learn a new job now.

On the third day of my training, sitting outside of a coffee shop in Malibu, my phone rang. It was the neuro-oncologist. I was in the middle of reviewing papers and charts with the person training me, and I apologized to her, excusing myself, saying I really needed to take this call.

"We think Emily could endure another short bit of radiation treatment," the doctor told me.

"Again? She's had it twice now already, although I know the last time was a small dose."

"It's honestly the best bet. There are no more chemotherapies appropriate for her to try. And I'm assuming you do not want to pursue surgery."

"You're right. No more surgery," I replied.

"Okay, I'll get you a meeting with the radiation oncologist next week."

With that, I took a deep breath and headed back to the table where my young colleague was sitting. I apologized again, and she asked if everything was all right.

"Fine," I responded. I couldn't tell this person, whom I had only met two days earlier and was promising that I'd do a great job, that no, I wasn't fine. My daughter has a brain tumor, and the doctor wants her to go through radiation treatment again, and my husband and I have major decisions to make. Instead, I put on that familiar fake smile and pretended to pay attention as we wrapped up the training session and took a tour of Malibu.

A week later, Dave and I sat in front of the radiation oncologist while Ryan sat at his desk in first grade and Emily attended her first week at her new special education classroom in junior high. This doctor, again, felt confident that radiation treatment was the way to go to treat these tumors that kept growing. He suggested just one week of low dose treatment. Quick, easy, painless.

"I don't think we should do it," I finally told Dave that night after the kids went to bed.

"What do you mean not do it?" He looked at me, confused.

"I don't want Emily to have radiation again," I said firmly, without emotion.

"What do you want to do then?"

"Nothing," I said. Why was he surprised? Why wasn't he nodding his head in agreement?

"Nothing? But radiation is easy, and she tolerates it well. If we do nothing the tumor will keep growing." He looked at me like I had two heads. I was shocked we weren't on the same page. I was ready to throw in the towel. I was so tired of treatments failing, of Emily feeling bad, I was just … broken down. But Dave clearly was not. He still wanted to fight.

I was at a crossroads. As much as I was ready to be done with treatment, I couldn't be the one to stand in the way when Dave, Emily's father, wanted to keep treating her. I couldn't have that on my conscience. And I didn't know what that would do to us in the end if I insisted she have no more treatment.

"Fine. We'll do the radiation," I finally relented after sorting through the thoughts in my head.

≈ 17 ≈

Chaos

Four weeks after I started my new job, Emily started her week-long radiation appointments. I was knee-deep into this new job, learning and doing at a rapid rate. This job was much more time-consuming than I was used to, and, although I was hoping for this sort of change, the timing could not have been worse. I didn't have vacation or sick leave to use for Emily's radiation appointments. But I was insistent that I was going to be the one to take her. Quite simply, I wanted to be there for her (for my sake as well as hers). I wanted to hold her hand as she fell asleep to the anesthesia, and I wanted to be the one who was there when she woke up from it, asking for juice. So I scheduled all my phone calls and meetings in the afternoons and would sit in the waiting room with my laptop, answering emails in the mornings while she was receiving treatment.

The first two days went fine. It was hectic, and I was exhausted from the schedule, from having the flu the week prior, and from my emotional state, but I managed it. On the third day, my brother Mike met me in the waiting room. He had a meeting in Denver and met us at the clinic for a quick visit. But the radiation clinic was running late. Hours late. I, consequently, broke down. I had meetings scheduled that afternoon that I was clearly going to miss. I was practically hyperventilating because I had never performed this poorly at a job before. Mike was stuck in a hard place trying to calm me down by offering me solutions, none of which seemed feasible. Instead I just sat there staring at my computer, watching emails and calendar requests pour in, and cried until Emily's name was finally called.

I sobbed that night to Dave, complaining about my job. "I can't handle it. Not with everything going on with Emily."

"Just quit," he calmly told me.

"I can't quit. We need the money. You know that. I just need to make it through this week," I rationalized more to myself than to Dave.

I squeaked out the rest of the week without losing my job or even getting reprimanded for the number of meetings I missed or moved around. More important, Emily got through the week. She handled these appointments without question but did complain more and more about the number of times she had to go to the doctor. "I know," I'd tell her, "but we go to the doctors to keep you healthy." She was getting to the age where an eye roll usually met my response to her complaints; she wasn't blindly believing everything I told her anymore. She had been through too much.

Thinking that I just needed to make it through that week was foolish. Although both kids were in school full-time, I could barely take the 10 minutes it took to drop Ryan off without getting interrupted by a phone call or supposedly urgent email. With my old job, I took advantage of being able to pause to attend to a scraped knee or chit-chat with another mom as I dropped my kids off at school. It may have been monotonous and boring, but I got to live the little life I had.

My days still started with walking Emily down the stairs at 5 a.m. It would then continue with getting her ready for the day (dressing, brushing teeth, eating breakfast, etc.) and checking to make sure Ryan was ready for the day. I'd get myself ready, get them to school, and then work. At the end of the day, after dinner and getting the kids ready for bed, including giving Emily a shower, I ended up back on the computer to tend to work that never seemed to go away. After two more nights filled with exhausted tears and late-night sessions on my computer, I threw in the towel. I tearfully told Dave that I really did need to quit. I was hating my life.

"Then quit. You are clearly over-stressed." He seemed very calm at the prospect of me quitting my job without having a new one lined up. I wasn't sure why—we needed my income in order to not live paycheck to paycheck.

"Maybe now we can seriously look at moving," was my response. Both Dave and I had fantasized about moving away from Colorado for some time now. I longed for a different environment—just something, anything, different. We talked about it without thinking we would really do it; after all, we had jobs and kids in school here, and my parents lived less than 10 minutes away. But we were also lonely for friends and a life.

"Can you talk to your boss about moving?" I asked. I was very serious now about the idea. Dave worked completely remotely—it didn't seem like it would matter where we lived.

"Okay, let's see what he says. So are you going to quit, then?"

"Yes. Are you sure it's okay?" I asked one more time, embarrassed that I thought I could handle a job like this and also praying that he was agreeable to the idea. "Maybe we can move to an area we can afford to live on with just your salary. Or I can just start looking for a new job wherever it is we end up."

"Yeah, you know I've been wanting to move too." My shoulders fell at his response; I was finally able to breathe again.

The next morning, I quit my job. Without a shred of remorse, I went on with my day wrapping up loose ends from a job I worked at for less than two months, lingered at the school drop off, and chatted with the other moms. That night, Dave and I poured over real estate listings in various states along the eastern seaboard. We were from the East Coast and longed for a similar environment for our kids to grow up in.

We researched different areas and were getting excited about the idea of such a big change and fresh start. We were hopeful we could move to an area where we could live comfortably with just one income and I could stay home and concentrate on the kids. I could be fully involved in their lives, their schooling, and not divide it up with work. I was finally excited about something.

But there were a few major things that hung us up. I was hesitant to leave my parents who had moved to Colorado nine years earlier. I assuaged my guilt with the knowledge Mike and Kim lived nearby. Plus, my parents had a pretty spectacular social life with a wide circle of friends. The other major obstacle was Medicaid. We couldn't afford Emily's healthcare without the help of this secondary insurance. Medicaid was a state-funded program, and the process and wait list for getting on the program varied by state. Finally, the thought that we were nuts for uprooting Emily from the care she'd been receiving at Children's Hospital since she was a baby came up often in our planning.

North Carolina kept coming up as a viable option during our research. One of the things that was on Dave's wish list was "no more snow," and North Carolina could come close to making that wish come true. However, I was not a fan of heat. I also was worried about moving to the South. The stereotypes about the area did not mesh with my political leanings, but I was trying to be open-minded. Helping with the open-mindedness was the cost of housing. We could afford to live there on just Dave's salary.

At Emily's next neuro-oncologist appointment, I brought up our idea to the doctor. "Dave and I are thinking about moving out of state."

"Oh, yeah?" The doctor looked at me, a bit surprised.

"Yeah. Can that be done? I mean, do people like us with kids who have such severe medical needs do that? Can we move?" I asked, feeling silly for having to ask permission, but really wanting to know if we were being outrageous to even think about moving.

The doctor laughed. "Yes! Of course. You are allowed to live your lives. You just need to find good care. Where are you moving?" he asked.

"We aren't sure yet but leaning toward North Carolina."

"Ah, my wife would love to move to North Carolina! If you end up there, you'd need to go to Duke University to get Emily's care. It's one of the top brain tumor medical centers in the nation. In fact, that's where we've sent her tumor biopsies to get examined."

I relayed all of this to Dave, started researching areas around Duke University and found that the area had everything we were looking for, especially a low cost of housing. I called their Department of Human Services and found that they had a similar Medicaid program—with no waiting period. With that, Dave met with his supervisors at work and got the blessing to move. The decision was made—we were going to move to North Carolina. And soon. Our savings account was dwindling quickly without my salary rolling in. I told my parents the next day, and although they were sad to see us go, as usual, they were supportive. My mom had seen how unhappy I was over the last few months and she was excited at the idea of me not having to work anymore.

In early October, my sister-in-law Kim, a realtor, put our house on the market. My parents offered to watch both kids while Dave and

I spent the weekend house hunting in Raleigh and getting a general feel for the area. One of our main priorities for our new house was a downstairs bedroom for Emily. No more stairs. She needed to be able to wake up independently in the morning, and I needed to sleep past 5 o'clock. There wasn't enough coffee in the world to keep waking up at that hour. Other than that, our priorities were to find a house in an area with excellent schools in a new neighborhood that had the promise of a lot of little kids for Ryan to play with. That weekend, we found our house in a small town outside of Raleigh that checked all the boxes, while only using Dave's salary to qualify for the mortgage. We signed the paperwork necessary to close on the house in early December.

Once back home, we let everyone know the news. We had a few goodbye get-togethers with friends, but otherwise it was an uneventful move. The oncologist contacted the doctor he wanted us to see at Duke University Hospital and sent over Emily's records. I got a copy of Emily's Individualized Education Plan to take to her new school. Ryan happily went along with the news, which wasn't surprising given his agreeable nature. Emily was a little more difficult just because she couldn't understand the timing (she started packing the moment we mentioned the move). And then she would forget that we were moving. I was over-the-moon excited. I had grand ideas of how our new life was going to look, and I looked forward to living it.

⇛ 18 ⇚

Welcome to NC

"What do you think, guys?" I asked Emily, now almost 13 years old, and Ryan, six years old, as we pulled into the driveway of our new home.

"It's nice," Emily said.

"I like it!" Ryan said.

We explored our new, empty house. Emily was happy to not have to use the stairs to get to and from her bedroom and Ryan loved that there was a dedicated playroom on the second floor and bedroom larger than the one he had in Colorado. Plus, we had a large yard, complete with trees, around which Sandy immediately ran laps. The next day, Friday, I registered the kids for school, and they started the following Monday.

Dave decided to paint the garage the day after our movers arrived. Meanwhile, I was walking around barefoot because I couldn't find the one pair of shoes I had with me and couldn't find the box that had all my other shoes packed away. I was in good spirits, though, because I had just hung up my winter coat, which felt heavy, and realized there were still rocks in the pocket to keep the coyotes away—hopefully I wouldn't need those anymore. I walked into the garage to ask Dave if maybe painting could wait when I saw a group of people walking down the street toward us, pulling a cooler behind them.

"Hi! We're the welcoming committee!" one of the guys said, laughing as he popped open the cooler and handed us a few bottles of beer. This group of neighbors introduced themselves, and we chatted for a while. We were all around the same age, and one was even from Connecticut. One couple mentioned that they had a son the same age as Emily. When they said we should get the kids together, I apologetically added that she had some cognitive and physical delays. There's never a great response to that comment, but I felt like I needed to put it out there. Like, don't expect them to hang out at the mall like most preteens. By the end of their impromptu visit, after sharing some laughs, we had an invitation to come over for drinks that weekend as well as an invitation for the family to go to a Christmas Eve bonfire at another's house. To top it off, we were all invited to a New Year's Eve party.

I was smitten after they left. Friends.

Ryan started at the local elementary school, which was just two minutes from our house. His school had a year-round calendar which meant he would go to school for nine weeks at a time and only have a three-week break in between sessions. After enduring long summer breaks for years, a year-round option sounded like heaven. Why couldn't we have had this for Emily all those years?! Emily's school, however, followed a traditional school calendar, still leaving us with the dreaded summers to fill for her. At least I didn't have to juggle a job with her routine now.

The weekend before school started, I walked with Ryan around the block hoping to see some kids outside playing. We saw evidence of kids—playsets, scooters on porches—but none were outside. A few hours later, I suggested we take another walk, but he said he didn't feel like it.

"Don't you want to see if there are any kids out playing? It will be nice to make some friends," I asked.

"No, it's okay. I can just play with Emily."

At this point, Ryan loved cars, anything superhero, Legos and video games, none of which Emily played with. In fact, I hadn't seen them play together in about a year. But that afternoon, Ryan busied himself in Emily's room. Emily still played with her baby dolls, and Ryan played along with her. He got the dog to join in and then an old game of playing "house" broke out. After one day of this (although nice to see and I wanted to encourage it), I knew Ryan would need his own set of friends, so I made him go for another walk with me. This time, success. We ran into two boys, exactly his age, riding bikes. He joined them that day, but he still made time to play with Emily when he was home. That weekend, at first lonely for Ryan, reignited his friendship with Emily. They continued to play together for many months moving forward.

Ryan now took a big yellow school bus to school—something he had never done before. It was incredibly hard for me to watch my six-year-old little boy, who only knew a small neighborhood school to which everybody walked, now go to a big school with buses and hundreds of kids. He was also the only one of us who left behind a close group of friends and an active life. Now, here he was walking up the steps to a bus to be dropped off at a school that he'd only seen for a few minutes the previous Friday and where he didn't know a soul. I was a wreck that day wondering how my sweet little bear was doing.

Emily, on the other hand, I had no doubts was doing just fine. She was confident and excited for this adventure. She had slowly grown back to her verbal self and was assertive in getting her needs met. I was introduced to her teacher the Friday I registered her for school and knew she was in great hands. Emily had also met some of her new classmates the day of registration and made a friend in one girl right off the bat. We were both excited when she got into the cab that morning at 6:30 (Emily received door-to-door transportation with her new school district).

Emily came home from school first and said it was fun. I had to email the teacher, of course, to get the actual details since I knew Emily couldn't remember. She concurred that she thought Emily had a great time. She said she was a joy to have in the class and continued her friendship with the girl she met on Friday. The teacher also said Emily fit right in. This, I knew, meant that the level and speed of instruction was perfect for Emily. Ryan came off the bus that afternoon with a smile on his face too.

While the kids were at school, Dave worked, and I stayed busy putting the house together and setting up all of Emily's many doctor's visits. I also started the process for Emily to receive services through the county, including Medicaid. We met with our newly assigned social worker, who helped us through the process during her home visit. She also suggested we get some home modifications done to better assist Emily. She put in a request for Emily to have grab bars installed in her bathroom, along with an extra handrail for our stairway in case Emily ever did have to go upstairs. Within weeks, these jobs were done. And not only did we now have an accessible house, the extra handrail was an actual *handrail*, not PVC piping.

Dave and I sat on the couch shortly after we moved and held hands. We knew we made the right decision moving here. Our kids were in good schools, we had big trees in our backyard, Ryan's shoes were muddy from playing in the woods, and we had plans for every weekend that month. We couldn't remember the last time we had plans for the weekend.

Once my parents learned that we would be in North Carolina in December, they made plans to come visit the week between Christmas and New Year's. This was a relief to me, as I was already having a difficult time leaving them—I was certain I wouldn't have been able to handle Christmas without them. We spent a good chunk of their visit checking out our new area, including lots of model homes in neighborhoods under construction. They were retired realtors, so I didn't think much of this pastime, and I enjoyed seeing how the homes were decorated. One of the nights of their visit, my dad asked Ryan what he thought of the new town he lived in. Ryan replied, "I like it. But who's the mayor of this place?"

My dad and I exchanged glances at my just six-year-old son before I interjected, "I'm not sure, but we can look it up. Why do you want to know?"

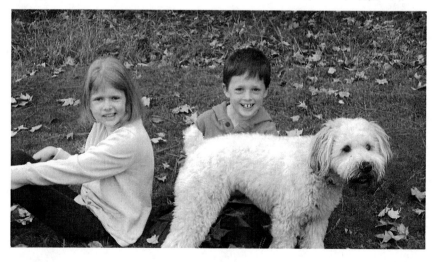

Emily and Ryan, with our dog, Sandy, during our first fall in North Carolina.

Ryan replied, "I want to write him a letter and ask to meet him."

With that, I looked up the mayor of our town and gave Ryan a piece of paper to write his letter. We stuck the letter in an envelope; Ryan put a stamp on it and put it in the mailbox. Three days later my phone rang, and the person on the other end of the line asked, "Is this the mother of Ryan?"

"Yes," I hesitantly answered.

"This is the mayor, and I'd like to set up a meeting to meet your son, if that's okay with you."

I laughed as we set up a meeting for Ryan to meet the mayor of our new town. A few days later, Ryan and I sat across from the mayor's desk in the fancy town hall. We got a tour of the building and a history of the town, and Ryan got to bang the gavel used at town council meetings. Eventually, the conversation turned to why we moved to North Carolina. When I got to the part that my daughter had some severe medical needs, and Duke was recommended as a place for treatment, he wanted to know more. So I talked about Emily, her diagnosis, her interests, and her limitations. He said, "I met with a man yesterday who is bringing a theater program to our town that is inclusive of all people, including those with disabilities—cognitive or physical."

The mayor then gave me information on the town's Civitan group, which was hosting this new theater program and asked me to attend the next meeting. A few weeks later I went to the meeting and met Alan, the amazing man bringing Together on Center Stage (TOCS) to town.

"TOCS," he explained, "is a performance art program for people regardless of their experience, abilities, or disabilities. It includes anyone from kids to adults, people who can walk or not, people who can talk or not—it doesn't matter. I create roles for them to perform on stage where they can showcase what they can do and get a round of applause."

"It sounds wonderful!" I exclaimed, but then the practiced excuses and reasons why this wouldn't work came out. "But my daughter has a right-side weakness—she doesn't use her right hand and has some balance issues. Plus, she has memory problems; she wouldn't be able to remember her lines."

"That's fine!" he said, adding, "Does she like to sing or dance?"

"She loves dancing," I let him know.

"Have her join the program! She can dance or do whatever else she wants to do."

And with that, Emily joined Together on Center Stage. We had been in North Carolina for just a few months and already felt like life was renewed. Dave and I had a set of friends that we felt comfortable around, laughing through our nights together, while all the neighborhood kids ran around every which way. Ryan was off playing with new friends and doing well in school. And let's not forget that he already met the mayor, which gave him his final stamp of approval for this new place we now called home. Even Emily had a new friend from school, with whom we now got together with at various parks and at our homes for playdates, and was involved in the community doing a theater program.

Emily had her first MRI at Duke within a month of moving to the area and met with her new neuro-oncologist after the scan. We were pleased to hear that the tumor was stable, but as we went through her medical history, her new doctor said he was concerned with the amount of radiation she endured. He thought it was too much for her young brain. We explained that, obviously, the doctors felt the need for treatment outweighed the possible effects from it at the time so we consented.

Next, we met with the neurologist to discuss Emily's seizure activity. After reviewing her medical history, he too asked, "Why so much radiation?"

"Well, that's what the doctors suggested as treatment. We really had no other options."

"It was too much."

"So I've heard."

The neurologist did a thorough exam of Emily's cognitive abilities while there as well, surprised at the level of reading she could do. "Yes, she's always been an excellent reader. If only she could remember what she read."

Miraculously, for some unknown reason, that February Emily's seizure activity stopped. She went a week with no seizure, then two weeks, then a month … still no seizure. The neurologist just said to keep her on the meds she was currently taking: "Let's not rock the boat." The other doctor we saw right away was the gastroenterologist.

Her Crohn's disease was never fully under control, and our move to North Carolina didn't change that. She had lost some weight and still had stomach pains, so keeping up with these appointments was a priority.

I kept so busy that winter and spring, I was just as tired at the end of the day as when I was working a job. In addition to attending and keeping track of all of Emily's medical appointments—seemingly endless that winter—I volunteered at Ryan's school one afternoon a week. I was enjoying my new full-time stay-at-home mom status.

But after those first few months, with the kids in school full-time, house set up, and doctors established, I found myself with a lot of spare time. I ended up finding some very part-time contract work to do from home to help keep me busy while earning mad cash that we could use for Christmas gifts that year.

That spring, when my parents returned for another visit, they asked to see a model house that they had seen on their previous visit because they decided to move here. This news relieved the guilt I felt about leaving them when we did, but it started a new worry that they wouldn't be as happy here as they were in Colorado. When they left, they had more than a hundred people attend their going-away party. Dave and I had a handful of friends who called to say goodbye. They had so much more to lose than we did. Thankfully, though, they also moved to a fun neighborhood and quickly made friends.

⇒ 19 ⇐

Aides

When I started the paperwork to get Emily on state-wide services in North Carolina, I was told that I was required to hire an aide to assist Emily. Just like when Emily's elementary school wanted to hire an aide all those years ago, I was totally against it. I was a stay-at-home mom now and fully able to take care of her. Plus, the aide would only work until 5 p.m. and Ryan didn't get home from school until 4:30 (whereas Emily got home at 2:15) so I knew having an aide wouldn't even give me much alone time with Ryan, which would have been helpful. I thought it was pointless.

My mom could not understand my anger. At all. "Let this person watch Emily while you run errands," she would say. "Go to the mall while the aide is with Emily."

The mall was a place I used to love. My love of shopping was a gift from my mother, who also relished the pastime. We spent hours at the mall together when I was young, trying on outfits and keeping our eye on all the sales. When I hit my preteen years, my mom would drop me off at the mall with my girlfriends where we would ooh and aah over the latest trends as well as boys passing by. And even when I was in college, Dave and I would spend Saturday afternoons at the mall shopping together. We joked that I had a dismal sense of direction but could easily get to any mall in the state. If I had to go somewhere new, I would ask, "What mall is it near?"

But over the last decade, my love of shopping all but disappeared. I no longer cared that my pants were dated, my shirt was from Walmart, or that there was an incredible sale going on at Gap. Perhaps I felt that way because it was too difficult to get to the mall by myself. Or that Emily had no patience for shopping so I rushed out as quickly as I could when we shopped together. Maybe it was because most of our extra funds paid for doctor appointments. Mostly, though, it was just no longer a priority.

I would cry on the phone to my mother, trying to explain why I didn't want an aide. "I don't want this person in my house. I'm home and Dave is home. It's ridiculous!"

My anger also came from the fact that I was forced to hire someone. I had very little control over my life with Emily, and this was one more strand taken away from me. This was just someone else I had to watch. The aide wasn't allowed to drive anywhere with Emily (per the state rules explained to me that afternoon) so even utilizing this person to take Emily to the library or McDonald's for an outing wasn't an option.

I was allowed several months to hire an aide, so I dragged my feet until the last possible minute. After interviewing four aides, I settled on one who could come to our house one or two afternoons a week. She was a soft-spoken, kind, older woman with whom Emily enjoyed speaking. I weeded out the woman who wanted to bring her toddler to our house while she took care of Emily, the one Emily couldn't understand, and the lady who wouldn't make eye contact with Emily.

A few weeks later, Emily's aide started her work. One or two afternoons a week, for two hours at a time, she came to our house. She would play board games with Emily, help Emily get out her dolls and dress them, and, sometimes, just sit with Emily while she watched TV. I would busy myself during this time with made-up chores a room away, so I could keep an ear on their conversations. Because I couldn't quite trust this person with Emily, I felt chained to the formal living room or dining room during the two hours the aide was here. It was not a productive time for me. However, I reluctantly admitted to Dave that Emily seemed to enjoy the company.

After about six months, she gave me her notice. She needed to stay home with her grandson who had just moved in with her. Although she did nothing to warrant my mistrust and the uncomfortable feeling I had with another person in my house, I waited the three months I was allowed before interviewing other aides.

A batch of questionable-quality people filed in and out of my house for the 10-minute interviews that consisted of questions like

"How long have you been a caregiver?" or questions concerning their scheduling needs. I'd watch the interactions between Emily and the stranger in my family room to gauge my feelings toward the person. There was no book or manual I could work from—I had to figure it out. In the end, I just listened to my gut, which wasn't always right.

The next aide I hired was a bit more energetic than the last one. She had great ideas for fun things she would do with Emily. The first few times she came over, they did a craft or two and then organized Emily's books. She and I spent a lot of time talking as well. The third time she came over, I hid in the other room. This woman could talk your ear off if you let her, and I wasn't in the mood for constant chatter. Plus, it annoyed Emily. The fourth time she came over, she spent the entire two hours dead-heading a plant on my patio. Emily watched TV in the family room while I hid in the front room. I called the agency that night and told them I would no longer need her services.

Now, I was thoroughly annoyed. I felt like a hostage in my own house when the required aide came to "help." So I continued the pattern of waiting three months before hiring a new person. Without fail, that aide would do something or nothing, as the case may be, before I let them go. One aide stole Ryan's birthday gift cards he received in the mail and left on the counter. One aide would sit on the couch while Emily played baby dolls in the other room. I had to explain the rules of Chutes and Ladders to one person, *repeatedly*, because she just could not grasp the concept of the game. A few here or there were good, quality caregivers, but they didn't last long due to the small paychecks. I was left feeling like this requirement was more of a punishment than a service. Poor Emily, though, had to deal with a constant string of people in and out of her life. Just when she would remember the aide's name, they would disappear.

Going through the journey of hiring aides we didn't want was worth it, though, considering it meant that Emily could get Medicaid as a secondary insurance. We endured the home visit and inspection from the social worker every three months as well as a nurse evaluation of Emily every six months. Each year I filled out the mountain of paperwork, and Emily was fully evaluated again by the caseworker and medical staff. After going through what it took for Emily to receive state-funded resources, I found it hard to believe the stories of people fraudulently obtaining services. Dave and I often joked that those stories must be wildly exaggerated, or the people obtaining services fraudulently were masterminds.

As we settled into our life in North Carolina, Emily's health started to stabilize. Although the Crohn's medication sometimes worked and sometimes didn't, the tumor hadn't grown for a while now, and she still wasn't having seizures. Dave and I never commented, "Boy, Emily sure is healthy these days!" Instead, we had fewer meltdowns surrounding the number of doctor appointments or feeling trapped at home because Emily was too ill to do anything. Dave continued working without interruption, I worked my small contract job while the kids were in school, and we had more normal conversations like "What do you feel like doing this weekend?" or "Let's plan a little getaway."

We were also more at ease socializing with our neighbors. Almost every weekend, we had a dinner at someone's house or people over to ours for drinks after Emily went to bed. In the summertime, we would meet at the neighborhood pool, which we could see from our house and was less than a one-minute walk away. Ryan would swim with his friends, Emily would draw pictures, and the adults would sit at a table with drinks and snacks. We'd bring Emily back home at 7 when she wanted to go to sleep, and sometimes we'd slip back to the pool to hang out a little more with neighbors. Dave and I would take turns opening the front door of our house to make sure she hadn't woken up. The fact that we were doing normal family things, things people did all summer long, summer after summer, wasn't lost on us. We relished it, appreciated it, and talked about it at home, late at night, away from our friends.

Our neighbors only knew that Emily had a brain tumor, but she was fine now, other than a cognitive and physical delay. They didn't know the horrors of surgeries, chemotherapy, or radiation or the damage all that treatment had caused. It wasn't that we kept it a secret; it was just something that wasn't brought up. We couldn't take the pity looks, even the well-meaning ones. We also didn't want to change the dynamics of our friendships. We wanted to be seen and thought of as *normal*. As we got close with a few people, we let them into our world, giving a little bit more of her history if asked. Otherwise, most people thought that all the medical issues were over and a distant part of her past.

⇒ 20 ⇐

Working

After working on my contract job for about six months, I received a phone call from my boss offering me a full-time job in the office. And, much to Dave's chagrin, I actually thought about it. Frankly, as much as I enjoyed being a stay-at-home mom, I was going stir crazy with the kids at school all day. When Ryan got home from school, he grabbed a snack and went outside to play with friends, not coming in until dinnertime. Emily came home from school exhausted, just wanting to sit and watch TV or color pictures. She had minimal doctor appointments to go to and no more weekly physical therapy visits. It was hard for me to go from 80 miles per hour, the speed I seemed to have traveled before our move, to the 20 miles per hour I was operating at now. I was antsy. But I also knew there was no way I could work full-time again, not with Emily's routine.

"No, I can't work that many hours. Sorry."

"You can! You really should think about it. The company is great—it's not a stressful place at all. Totally family friendly." Bob, my boss, was working hard to convince me to take the position.

"Could I work from home?" I couldn't believe I was contemplating this job.

"Not initially, but yeah, we can work towards that," he compromised.

"I have a daughter with special needs. I'm not the most reliable person—if things come up, she's my priority." Now I was trying to talk him out of wanting to hire me.

"You'll be fine. It's a great place to work." Bob went on to tell me exactly where the office was—just 20 minutes from my house—and the salary—more than I had made in any other job.

"Let me talk with Dave. I'll call you back."

I took all the notes I had written during my phone call with Bob and walked upstairs to Dave's office. "Hey," I said. "You'll never guess what just happened." I then relayed the whole conversation. He responded as he usually does in these situations, stating whatever I wanted to do would be fine with him, but reminded me how difficult it was to manage work with Emily and that one of the reasons we moved here was so that I wouldn't have to work. I countered with my boredom, the fact that the kids were in school longer here, Em had fewer appointments, and the money was really good.

Although leaving my job in Colorado was easy, I had a difficult time grasping the idea that I no longer had my own salary. I felt that I lost a piece of independence when I stopped working. More than the independence that I felt I lost, though, we weren't saving as much as we used to when I worked, and that scared me.

Emily would most likely live with us for the rest of her life. We didn't fully think about what life would truly look like having her in our house the rest of our lives, as we still lived day to day, but we knew that was our reality. She wasn't going anywhere. We needed to be able to afford not only to take care of us during our retirement but to take care of her for the rest of *her* life.

I called Bob back and hashed out a deal. Instead of negotiating my salary, I negotiated my schedule. I would accept the full-time position and work in the office for the first three weeks. After that, I'd work Fridays from home for another few weeks, and then, add another day from home. Hopefully, at some point, I would work fully from home.

A week later I started my new job in this corporate office. Not only was I nervous about working in general, I was worried about working at a for-profit company. The last few times I got a job in the corporate world, it lasted mere weeks. Those first few weeks on the job did me in. Leaving in the morning was fine. I got up at my usual 5:45 to dress Emily, who was already awake and watching TV in the family room. I made us breakfast, then brushed Emily's teeth and laid out her pills. I put her lunch, made the night before, in her book bag, and when Sandy started barking at 6:40, I walked Emily outside to the cab that had just pulled up. By this time, Ryan was awake. He got up and dressed himself before coming downstairs. I made sure he was eating before I hopped in the shower and got dressed for work. I came downstairs in time to see Ryan off to the bus stop at 7:30. I was usually able to make it to my desk on time at 8.

Coming home, however, was a different story. By 5, I was exhausted—like, Emily as a baby exhausted. My brain was on the entire time I was at work, and the pace was quick. The office was regimented. Everyone, it seemed, was at their desk at 8 a.m. and didn't get up until their one-hour break for lunch at noon. They didn't leave their desks again until exactly 5 p.m. I was not used to the rigidness of the day—by either my home standards or my previous work standards. There was a level of trusted autonomy I, apparently, took for granted in my previous roles. By the time I walked through the door at 5:30 p.m., I was ravenous and spent. I didn't have the energy to keep up with the kids' excitement as they told me about their days. I certainly didn't have it in me to make dinner—something I had always done. "It'll be fine once I get to work from home," I told Dave, hoping I was right.

I mustered up all the energy I could to get through those first several weeks of work, certainly appreciating when the weekends arrived. Work in this corporate office was all business. There was no getting to know your coworkers; it was just me sitting in front of my computer sitting next to someone else sitting in front of their computer. Time at the proverbial "water cooler" was not a thing here. The upside was that I did not need to struggle with if or what I told colleagues about Emily. I didn't know anything about anybody, and all they knew about me was my email address and that I managed the surveys.

Finally, the time came for me to work just three days in the office and two days at home. Between the two days at home and me growing into the routine, I was feeling more comfortable in my role as a working mom. I was making it work, with the help of Dave. He picked up the slack at home by being there when the kids came home from school, doing the laundry, and sometimes getting dinner together (i.e., ordering take out). And we would both pop open a beer or make a gin and tonic on Friday nights feeling like we deserved the wind-down it provided.

Around this same time, Emily was in her first Together on Center Stage production. She had been going to rehearsals two times a week for several months. A week in, Emily came home with instructions to pick out her favorite song. A week after that, Emily was to write lines about the character she chose to be—a dancing chef. I had no idea where this was going but I did not have high hopes for it.

During the first few weeks of rehearsal, I sat outside the theater, on the floor in the hallway eavesdropping, knowing Emily wouldn't be able to recall what she did. And as I sat there, I was blown away by the instruction, compassion, and talent coming out of that room. I still had no idea how the show would play out, since each participant chose their own character and wrote their own lines. A gutsy move with this population. I was just thankful that Emily had a safe and caring environment in which to sing and dance her heart out.

On the Friday night of her first show, Dave, Ryan, and I sat in the second row of the new theater in town, which had a stage and more than 180 seats. We spied a few neighbors and their families in the sold-out audience and waved. Right on time, the curtain rose, and there was Emily, sitting with 10 new friends and some volunteers. She had a chef hat and an apron on, dressed for the part. The show opened with everyone singing the TOCS song, including dance moves and hand gestures that Emily, amazingly, did right in time with everyone else. Then, a boy about her age slowly rose and walked to a chair in the middle of the stage. He carefully sat down and a volunteer placed a guitar in his hands and put the strap around his neck. He clearly had movement issues and difficulty speaking, but with the lyrics to Journey's "Don't Stop Believin'" shown on a screen behind him, the entire audience sang along with him as he crushed it on the guitar. At the end of the song, the volunteer took the guitar from him allowing him to take a bow. The entire audience jumped to their feet applauding and screaming his name and his smile lit up that room more than any spotlight. My tears started flowing and didn't stop until the show was over. Each participant had their turn. Emily got up at the appropriate time (thanks to a cue from a volunteer) and walked up to the microphone. She spoke her lines, which were sitting on a music stand in front of her, then danced like she'd never danced before. The audience went wild, including me and Dave, although our hearts stopped a few times thinking she was going to dance right off the stage. Our neighbors came up to us after the show, wiping away their tears, feeling the same way I did. It's all any parent wants—their child to be happy and appreciated.

When Emily was home from school in the summer, she attended a week-long overnight camp in the area that we found out about from a friend of Emily's from school.. She happily went away for four nights to this specialized camp while Dave, Ryan and I stayed home doing things like taking long walks in the evening and dining out. It was amazing how at ease I felt dropping her off at these specialized camps now. I almost felt like Emily was in better hands there, with doctors and nurses as counselors, than in my care. It helped that Emily loved her independence and relished the time away from us. Ryan was still in school, so I was able to easily go into the office while Emily was away. When she wasn't in overnight camp, there were other specialized day camps in our new area she attended to whittle away her summer days.

Ryan, however, was a little disappointed our first summer in North Carolina because a group of our friends, who had kids with whom Ryan was friends, had planned a vacation together on the coast, and we were not going. We were invited and even thought about it for a few days, but the reality of what the week would really look like traveling with Emily made us turn down the trip. We knew we wouldn't be able to be on the beach all day or do the trips to the lighthouse or even have dinner out if it were to run past 7 p.m. One of us would always be staying back with Emily or tending to her. It was easier to decline than to bear witness to everyone else being carefree while we were anything but. We also didn't want to slow down any of our friends' activities—knowing they, too, would not want us to feel left out. Of course, Ryan didn't understand this. He just knew that his friends were all going to the beach without him. We were once again thankful for Ryan's year-round school calendar. He didn't have much time to pout since school quickly started and soon summer vacations would become distant memories.

By the end of the summer I still hadn't gotten my full remote status at work, but that was about to change. Bob, my supervisor and the person who hired me, got laid off. The company got reorganized, and I was given all his duties (on top of my own) without a raise or promotion. This left a deep wound as I felt both overwhelmed and taken for a ride. I called Dave from work and shakily told him the news, trying hard to fight back the tears.

"Quit," he offered. "You can find something else. And isn't this why we came here? So you wouldn't have to work?" This was the first, of many, many times, Dave told me to quit this job.

I knew he was right, but the lure of someday working from home full-time, as well as the paychecks, kept me there. When I brought up the injustice I felt to my new supervisor, he said he understood, but his hands were tied. And then I asked about working from home five days a week. He came back to me the next day and said we had a deal.

Now things were really falling into place with me at home full-time, taking away some of the sting of not getting a promotion. Emily, though, had struggled with her Crohn's disease and was now on a medication that required frequent lab draws. She ended up needing a mediport surgically implanted to help with the lab draws since her veins were so shot. She also started having occasional seizures. Not a lot—roughly one seizure every few weeks—but enough for me to fear that the good times might end. Again.

When the worry would start to rise, I would tell myself that Emily was still a happy, sassy girl. Ryan was doing well in school and enjoyed good friendships. Dave and I had friends and a much-needed social life. I could earn a paycheck without leaving my house. I had the flexibility to take Emily to a doctor's appointment without missing an entire afternoon of work. Ryan would always see me when he got home from school. All the while, we were building up our savings account again. These were the things that I prioritized in my life.

During one of the summer breaks, Emily got a job at a place that only hires adults with disabilities. They do all sorts of jobs for companies with whom they contract, and for one particular contract, they hired high-school-aged people. I heard about this like I did with most activities for Emily: from other parents of kids with special needs. I dropped Emily off at 9 each morning for two weeks, and she folded towels during her four-hour shifts, taking a short break for lunch. Usually, I would pick her up and she would exclaim, "Phew, that was a lot of work!" On the last day I picked her up and she said, "A boy kissed me!"

"Um, what?" I asked, trying to be cool.

"Yup. Right here." She pointed to her cheek.

"Well … what happened?" I asked, fearful something bad had occurred.

"I was talking to a boy and he said I was cute and kissed me!" I glanced at her while driving down the road. She was beaming.

"What boy was it?"

"I don't know." Stupid memory. Of all the things to forget.

"How do you feel about the boy kissing you?" I asked.

"Nice. But don't tell Dad," she said.

"Don't tell Dad a boy kissed you?"

"Yes, don't tell Dad a boy kissed me."

"Okay. I won't say anything."

"Promise you won't tell Dad."

"I promise."

"Don't tell Dad a boy kissed me."

"Em, I won't say anything to Dad."

She proceeded to tell me not to tell Dave a boy kissed her the entire 30-minute drive home, and I repeatedly told her I wouldn't say anything. We finally got home and walked into the kitchen, where Dave was standing, and Emily announced, "A boy kissed me!"

I sighed audibly.

Dave asked, "A boy *kissed* you?" then turned to me with wide eyes.

"Yup!"

Dave was still looking at me. I just smiled and shrugged. I was curious how Dave was going to react to this news. By now, I was fine because she was so happy … plus it was the last day of work; she wouldn't be going back.

"Did you like it?" he asked her.

"Yes. I can't believe a boy kissed me!" she said again.

We all laughed, Dave included.

Later, he told me, "She's a teenager. It's actually nice to see something normal happen to her and for her to have a normal reaction." God help us.

When Emily was 15 years old, she started attending the local high school which was less than five minutes from our house. This is the school that she would attend for seven years since North Carolina allows children like Emily to remain in public schools until they are 22 years old. Thankfully, Emily's teacher in her high school classroom was a wonderful fit for her, and I was happy she would spend so much time under her guidance. Much like Emily's kindergarten teacher, she was compassionate yet didn't take any nonsense from the students. But I think I loved this teacher the most because she let me host birthday parties for Emily in her classroom.

It was getting harder and harder to celebrate Emily's birthday. She still expected parties like she had when she was young … stuck at seven years old since the stroke. She still played with dolls and the Wii. She still colored rainbows and butterflies and enjoyed her cartoons. And for birthday parties, she expected all her friends (the ones that she remembered from that age), balloons, streamers, and pin the tail on the donkey. But she was well into her teens now, and frankly, I couldn't fathom hosting yet another birthday party. When I asked her teacher if I could bring cake to the class on her birthday, she said yes. And then I took it a step further and asked, "Can I also bring crafts for all the kids to do and call it a party?"

"That would be fantastic!" was her teacher's response.

So, every year starting in high school, we held Emily's birthday party in her classroom. I would go in with cake and the craft and special paper plates that Emily picked out the week before. All her classmates plus usually some other staff who knew Emily, like the resource officer and maintenance man, came to wish Emily well, sing happy birthday to her, and have a slice of cake.

≋ 21 ≋

The Tumor. Again

The fall before Emily had her 16th birthday, she had a routine MRI. By now, she was enduring these MRIs every six months with no anesthesia. She would lie in the giant tube with headphones playing music as the machine took images, sounds of banging and rattling filling the room. I sat in the room with her now, plugs in my ears, reading a book. After 20 minutes in the tube, the tech would slide her out and put contrast dye in the IV placed in her arm. Then it was back in the tube for another 20 minutes of images and banging.

The worst part of MRI days was getting the IV placed. Although she had a mediport, it was finicky and Emily's veins were shot. It usually took multiple tries and, ultimately, an ultrasound machine to help guide the nurse to a workable vein. And Emily hated every minute of it. She was tired of waiting rooms and tired of the long procedures. She especially hated "pokes," her term for the needle stick. We learned not to talk about upcoming doctor's appointments in front of her—it caused immediate tears and anxiety. She would repeat, as she often does due to her short-term memory loss, "I don't want to go to the doctor." Her eyes would water, and her lower lip would jut out and tremble; her face resembled a toddler's face when upset. And I crumbled from a broken heart every time this happened.

I learned to only tell Emily she had a doctor's appointment on the day of, sometimes waiting until I loaded her into the car, feeling like a kidnapper. I wanted to avoid The Face. Her teacher found this out as well, after telling Emily that I was picking her up early from school one day because she had a doctor's appointment. Emily cried from 9 a.m. until I picked her up at noon. Her teacher told me she would never do that again.

Even though we hadn't heard the words *the tumor is growing* in several years, I didn't register shock or surprise when the neuro-oncologist muttered that dreaded phrase at this routine MRI visit, pointing at the films of Emily's brain. I had never let it go—the threat of the tumor growing was always looming in the background. Waiting.

"I'm going to need a few days to come up a with a treatment plan," the doctor said.

"We're scheduled to leave on a seven-day cruise tomorrow. We won't have consistent service. Should we cancel?" I asked calmly. I'd accepted our fate.

"No! That's wonderful! You go and enjoy the trip. I'll call you the following week."

I called Dave when we got in the car like I always did on MRI days. All I said was, "Growing."

"Growing?"

"Yes," I responded.

He paused, then asked, "Are you all right?"

"Yup. I'll see you in a little bit," I said and got off the phone.

I drove home the rest of the way in silence. Emily nodded off in the seat next to me. I tried to let numbness wash over me but couldn't stop the thoughts from forming. *Is there any treatment left? Would Dave and I consent to the treatment if there is a viable option? Are we going to be on the same page regarding her treatment? If we don't treat her, how long will she live? Will she suffer? If we do treat her, what will she suffer from the side effects? What would this do to Ryan? What would this do to us?*

I got home and said hello to Dave and Ryan. We got Emily settled drawing pictures on the kitchen table, and Dave and I went upstairs to talk.

"All he said was that it was growing, and he needed a few days to figure out a treatment plan," I relayed to Dave.

"Did you tell him about the trip?" he asked.

"Yeah, he was like *go—have a good time.* Right, like that's possible," I sighed. "What do you want to do? Do you still want to go?" We were planning on leaving at 4 the next morning to drive more than 12 hours to Miami. Once there, we were to board a cruise ship and meet up with our friends, Steve, Sonja and their girls, who were coming in from Colorado. I, for one, no longer had any desire to go on this trip.

"Yeah, I want to go. You're sure it's okay to go? She's okay?" he asked. The last cruise we took was successful, giving us so many happy memories.

"Yes. It's a small growth. I told the doctor we'd be gone and on a cruise ship for a week. He thought it was fine."

"We might as well go, then. At least we can all have a good time for a little while."

I couldn't think of an argument that wasn't just "I want to sit at home and sulk." Plus, I didn't want to ruin the trip for Ryan. So I continued the laundry and packing. But I was not excited. Nothing was exciting anymore. The thought of the tumor growing, once again, played like a movie in the front of my brain.

The good news was that I barely remembered the 12-hour car ride to Miami the next morning. We had a fun reunion with our friends as we waited to board the giant ship and settled into our cabins. I quickly barricaded both doorways in the kids' cabin, remembering the fiasco from last time. And that evening at dinner, we told our friends about Emily's tumor growing yet again, but we didn't talk about it after that. We didn't get too deep that entire week with our friends, conversations staying on the surface. I don't know if it was because we weren't ready to talk about it or if too much time and distance had passed between us.

We spent a lot of time on the boat and Dave was growing more tense as the week progressed, snapping at one point as we were wandering aimlessly in search of a restaurant. I, too, was growing more agitated with people. *Stop taking the fucking elevators!* I wanted to shout to the hordes of people jammed in as I waited for another crowded elevator that might have room for me and Emily. I vowed to never take a cruise again.

By the time we got home, I was ready to just deal with this tumor and get on with life. Dave and I couldn't talk about the upcoming discussions we were going to be having with the doctor while on vacation because we never discussed these things in front of the kids. We did not have a lot of alone time that week. But after a week of not discussing it, it just seemed easier to keep not discussing it.

A few days after we returned, we went, as if on a death march, to the neuro-oncologist's office to talk about Emily's tumor growth. I knew that chemotherapy was no longer an option from our previous oncologist. It had been pointed out several times that she already endured too much radiation. The only other cancer treatment left that we knew of was surgery to debulk the tumor. Dave and I long ago agreed that she would never endure a craniotomy again. So we walked into the doctor's office with our dukes up, ready to fight against the suggestion of surgery, the only option left, it seemed.

We were shocked, then, when the doctor recommended putting her on a type of chemotherapy in pill form that we could give her at home for a little more than a year, agreeing the tumor was in a spot that was too risky for surgery. "What?" I asked, completely blindsided by his suggestion of more chemotherapy.

"Yes, it's just a pill to give her at home. The downside," he said, "is that it has demonstrated stabilizing patients only 50 percent of the time. We wouldn't expect it to shrink the tumor, but hopefully it would stop it from growing. The upside—it's easy to administer and doesn't have many side effects." The side effects, he went on to explain, were low blood counts and immune system deficiency. That was old news to us and manageable. She would need to have her labs pulled often, but other than that, just another pill in her pill box. It was amazing how much advancement there had been in chemotherapies in such a short period of time.

"Really? That's it, just a pill?" Dave asked, shrugging his shoulders, smiling.

"That's it," the doctor replied.

I wasn't smiling or impressed with the easiness of it all. Nothing about this was easy. I wasn't falling for that anymore. But I was intrigued by just a pill. No nausea or hair falling out. No hospital visits. Just a pill. Not great odds at working but better than doing nothing.

Dave was clearly on board for Emily to take the pill form chemotherapy. After being prepared for a possible end, you grasp at things. It did seem too easy not to try. I nodded my consent to the pill.

Emily started taking the new white pill in her pill box on the appropriate days. Weeks went by and we didn't notice any change or effect from the pill. She continued to go to school. I worked full-time from home, Dave worked from home, traveling occasionally, and

Ryan was busy with school and his social life. Life was seemingly routine, albeit with an undercurrent of terror knowing the tumor had grown again.

I had no one to tell at work since barely anyone knew that I had a daughter, never mind one with medical needs. Dave didn't mention anything to his colleagues, either, as he always kept this information close to the cuff. We didn't tell Ryan all the details, other than she was on a new medicine that might make her feel bad, because we never told him these things. He was too young. We told only a few close friends, Emily's teacher, and my family. That was it. Most of the people in our lives did not know. The struggle to fit in, to not attract attention, to want a normal life, made us stay quiet.

Our days looked like our days before chemotherapy, except the lab results were never great. Her platelet counts always seemed to be low. The first time the labs came back, they were so low she needed to have a blood transfusion. It was a several-hours-long procedure that I sat through, unprepared for how long it was going to take.

For the first time, I grew more frustrated that I was missing work than the fact that my daughter was sick and needing blood. I had already been sneaking away time and time again for labs, pharmacy pick-ups, and doctor appointments over the last several months. Now I was annoyed at missing another full afternoon. Maybe I wouldn't have felt so guilty about the amount of work I was missing and the rearrangements in my schedule if I told my supervisors and colleagues about Emily's condition. But I was scared that if I told them about my situation, I would be viewed as a weak link—one they should let go. The company was quick to "lay off" people. How different the competitive, for-profit arena felt compared to the non-profit environments I worked in previously.

About a month later, as I was getting Emily undressed for a shower, I noticed a line of red dots under her skin on her chest. I texted the oncologist and described this rash. He told me I had to immediately get her labs drawn. An hour later, after labs were drawn and results were read, he said to bring her straight to the clinic for another transfusion. This time I packed my work computer and plenty of paper and markers for Emily, acting like a soldier gearing up for her next mission. The clinic was empty, as it was President's Day, and we had the lone nurse there to ourselves. It took about an hour for the nurse and the extra staff she called in to get an IV placed, using an ultrasound machine to find a willing vein. Emily was miserable through it all, no longer the smiling, dancing girl joking with medical staff. Finally, the hours-long transfusion could start.

At 8 p.m., the nurse apologized repeatedly while telling me that she had to send us down to the E.R. to get admitted for the rest of Emily's transfusion. The clinic needed to close, and Emily still had a few hours left of the procedure. Other than the fact that I had to log off my computer in order to relocate, I didn't understand why she was so apologetic until we got down to the Emergency Room and saw that it was packed full of people. However, our escort flagged a triage nurse and explained that Emily was undergoing chemotherapy and was in the middle of her transfusion, which got us promptly checked in and placed in a room, separate from the risk of infection lingering in the waiting room. I thought we were saved, except that the wait for the nurse to start the transfusion was another hour or so due to how busy they were. We didn't leave the Emergency Room until 1 a.m., fully understanding why the nurse apologized over and over again.

Another month went by, this time without issue. Emily was able to attend the first prom-like dance for people with special needs in the town. Several groups worked together to put on this free event, which included a red carpet for the attendees to walk down as they entered the dance floor. My mom and I took on the task of taking Emily shopping for a prom dress. It wasn't an easy one—besides the effort of getting Emily changed and unchanged to try on the dresses, clothes do not fit her the way clothing fits most people. Her right-side weakness causes her right shoulder to droop down, and her right leg is shorter than her left leg, making her hips a bit twisted. Even with these challenges, though, Emily's mood was soaring. She loved looking at all the dresses and trying them on. To her, they were all pretty, and each one made her look beautiful. I, on the other hand, was growing frustrated, both from the physical exhaustion of dressing and undressing her with each dress we tried on as well as with the fit of the dresses. I had to restrain myself several times from tearfully throwing in the towel. None of the dresses fit her appropriately. At one point I said to her, "Emily, this doesn't have to be so frustrating."

"I'm not frustrated," she said, smiling.

And she wasn't. I took my cue from her and her incredible spirit, took a deep breath, and relaxed. Finally, at the end of that long day, we found a dress that fit her well. She beamed at herself in the mirror, remarking, "I look so pretty!"

"You look gorgeous, Em." And she did.

I got her dressed the night of the dance. She wore a white tea-length dress with brightly colored flowers and a skirt that swooshed when she walked. She picked out jewelry to wear and looked in the mirror, grinning from ear to ear. After a million pictures were taken, we went to the dance. Emily walked down the red carpet, and once she heard the music, she was dancing. There was no stopping her. I stayed about a foot away from her during the night so I could right her when her balance drifted and to shield her from some of the wilder dancers there that evening. The feeling I had when I sat with Emily on the jungle gym when she was a preschooler, with all the other moms on the park benches, came flooding back to me, although this time, I'm sure the moms at this dance had an understanding of me being in the middle of the dance floor with the young participants.

She continued to dance the night away. All the way until 7:40. At that point, Emily turned to me mid-dance and said, "I need to go home. I'm tired." So I drove this exhausted girl home while she sat in the passenger seat next to me flipping through all the pictures I had taken on my phone, just like any other teen girl would do after a dance.

On the Sunday morning of Memorial Day weekend, a few weeks later, I noticed that Emily's legs were puffy. This had happened more and more over the last few weeks. But it came and went and never got too alarming. This time, though, in addition to the puffy lower legs, there were purple spots, much like the rash she had on her chest a month ago. I called the oncologist and explained the rash. I assumed he would say that she needed labs drawn and a transfusion. Instead, he asked that we FaceTime so he could see the rash over the phone. Ever so grateful for technology and his availability, I connected for a video chat.

After the video chat, the doctor concluded it was a different rash. She needed labs drawn but could wait until the next day to get them. A little bit later Emily complained of her stomach hurting. This was not uncommon, because of the Crohn's disease, but this too

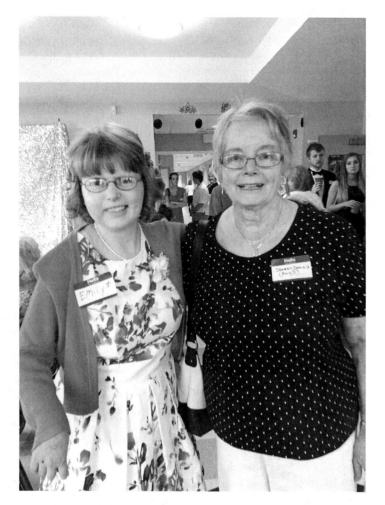

Emily and Nana at Emily's prom.

seemed to be a different kind of pain. Only after 10 minutes did the screaming stop.

Two hours later, she had another writhing, screaming session. I texted the oncologist to update him on Emily's pain. He relayed that he did not think it was related to the chemotherapy, but I should get in contact with her GI doctor if it persisted. I couldn't easily text the GI doctor like I could the oncologist and didn't feel like explaining this whole bit to the on-call doctor who knew nothing of her complicated case. At a loss for anything else to do to get her comfortable, I brought her to her bed to lie down. We were supposed to go to a neighbor's house for a barbecue that evening, so I told Dave to just go with Ryan while I stayed home with Emily. I struggled with the idea of bringing her to the Emergency Room. It's just a stomachache. But it was a severe one, I wrestled with myself. And why do these things always happen on a holiday weekend?

Later that night, after the boys returned from the barbecue, Emily screamed again. "That's it. I need to take her, don't I?" I asked Dave. He was always my sounding board.

When he nodded his head, I packed my bag with a change of clothing for both of us, along with my iPad and some paper and markers for Emily. We made the 40-minute drive to Duke's Emergency Room where, again, it was crowded. Thankfully, her chemotherapy status gave us priority in the crowded waiting room. We didn't even make it to the chairs before they called her back to triage.

By now it was midnight. I was exhausted, and Emily was starting another screaming fit. As sorry as I was for Emily, I said a little thank you to the gods who were listening that the staff could witness what I was trying not so successfully to explain. The doctors rushed to the room and examined her, got an IV placed, pulled some labs and gave her morphine which caused her to drift off to sleep, at which point I slouched over in the hard-plastic chair and couldn't stop myself from nodding off. At 2 a.m. the doctor came back in and said, "I think she has what is called Henoch-Schonlein purpura, or HSP for short. That purpura rash on her legs is very common with this disease, and it affects the intestines as well. She might have some kidney issues with it, which is common." Great, another line in her medical chart.

I only nodded; extreme fatigue had set in for me.

"We're going to admit her to run some more tests and to help her manage her pain. But there's no treatment to make it go away—it will, unfortunately, just need to run its course."

Emily was comfortably sleeping with the morphine rushing through her veins. I went back to nodding off in the hard-plastic chair. I couldn't form any questions to ask the doctor. My brain just wasn't comprehending at that hour. Finally, at 4 a.m., we were wheeled to an inpatient room in the hospital for our stay. I was so tired, all I could think about was the pleather recliner next to Emily's bed. It looked like a lush, king-size mattress compared to the hard-plastic chair in the Emergency Room.

Emily was so unwell she didn't even balk at the prospect of staying overnight in the hospital. She was given more morphine because the pain, along with the screaming, had come back. I sent Dave a text letting him know that we were admitted to the hospital and I would call him after morning rounds.

The doctor came to see us early that morning and explained what the ER doctor had already explained to us. They were going to run tests and keep an eye on Emily's kidney function since that could be affected with this disease, but otherwise, they were there to manage her pain. I relayed all of this to Dave and added, "Hopefully we can go home tonight or tomorrow. Since there's no treatment I can't imagine we'll be here long." I'm not sure how I could be so optimistic after all this time. And as usual, the goal for hospital stays became coming home, the work toward that goal starting as soon as she was admitted.

One night turned into nine long nights. Emily's pain was so severe that they gave her a push-button morphine pump. I learned, from doctors and the Internet, that HSP can last as long as six weeks and have recurrences throughout life. Unsurprisingly, Emily's oncologist told me he was stopping the chemotherapy while she was sick. He asked that we meet in a few weeks to touch base.

After the first day, Dave brought in my laptop so I could work during Emily's morphine stupors. Ryan was old enough now that we could talk on the phone in the evenings. He told me about his school days, and I reminded him to do his homework. He let it slip that "Dad and I don't eat dinner until eight o'clock at night! And we eat on the couch!" I just laughed at how animated he was and shook my head. I knew the only thing Dave made for dinner was spaghetti and the thought of them eating that on my light beige couch made me cringe.

This was a far cry from our usual routine. On most nights we ate dinner by 5:30. Way too early for Dave and Ryan, they'd complain. But Emily has limited things she thinks about, and dinner is one of them. When she gets home from school at 2:15 she asks what's for dinner. She'll ask three more times by 4. She'll have made a list of dinner ideas, even if I already have dinner planned out. By 4:30 she has set the table, complete with water glasses. She'll even have pulled out items from the pantry so I can start cooking. And I finally do because I can't stand the questions, the comments, and the talk about dinner anymore. I just want it over with. So we eat early and Emily is satisfied.

The older Ryan got, the easier it became to be away from him practically and logistically. The strong ache in my heart, however, remained the same. The problem with this hospital stay was that I kept thinking we'd be going home the next day. But the next day would come, and the doctor would say no, or Emily would scream all day in pain, and I'd know we were there another night. But each day I had hope. And this hope led me to tell my friends, Dave and Ryan included, not to visit. "I think we might be going home today or tomorrow. No need to come!" I made a mental note for future hospital stays to not use the hope of leaving the next day as a reason for people to not visit. Visits were a wonderful distraction from mundane hospital life, and we missed out on those that long stay.

≋ 22 ≋

Decisions

Once Emily recovered and was discharged from the hospital, we had a meeting to talk with the oncologist about her chemotherapy, which was stopped after her HSP diagnosis. In preparation for our meeting, Dave and I did a lot of talking. We started taking walks around the block by ourselves, leaving the kids home alone so we could talk without interruptions. During these walks, we decided not to continue treatment for Emily. This time it was an idea that Dave brought up. The doctor had already discontinued her chemotherapy while Emily was in the hospital, but we were concerned he would start it up again now that she was feeling better. Once Dave mentioned that he was no longer comfortable with the medicine, resulting in constant hospital visits and her feeling miserable—both emotionally and physically—a weight lifted off my shoulders. We were finally on the same page. The thoughts of stopping her treatment had rumbled in the back of my brain ever since I first thought about it years ago. We didn't want to see her suffer anymore. Sixteen years of hell was enough. We continued to talk about this, the ramifications of it, the what-ifs. We talked through many scenarios and still decided no treatment was her best option. We are true believers in quality of life, and Emily was suffering too much from the treatments. She was becoming ... not Emily.

We had our scheduled conference call with the doctor, and he spoke first. "Emily can't be on that chemotherapy anymore. She needed too many transfusions and got too sick on it. I've ended the prescription altogether. I'd like to have you speak with the neurosurgeon."

"We don't want to do surgery." I was barely audible when I said these words.

"What? I don't think you should make that decision without speaking to the surgeon." The doctor was pleading with us now. We understood it was his job to do everything medically possible to save Emily's life. The struggle came from believing it was our job to give Emily a *happy* life. We concluded the call with the doctor, after he suggested, again, we talk to a surgeon because that was the only viable treatment option left, and we declined, again.

Two days later, back into my reality of work emails, Emily's same, constant routine, Ryan in the midst of pre-teen hormones, and the knowledge that we made the decision to stop treating Emily's tumor floating in my head, I broke. Emotions flowed out of me like a river with a broken dam. I sat with Dave one night on our back porch. We were talking about Emily's future, like we often did at that time, and I started crying. I complained that I'd been bathing, dressing, and feeding her for 16 years now, and I would have to for the rest of her life. I complained that we had to get a babysitter for our almost-adult daughter if we needed to leave the house. Then I felt the guilt, because Emily always smiled and was quick with a back rub and an *I love you*. I wondered if my decision to stop her treatment was selfish. The lines got blurred as to what was best for *her* to live a quality life and for *me* to live a quality life. And then I was wailing. Emotions were running through me like an electrical current. I couldn't imagine her leaving us, yet I couldn't imagine taking care of her much longer. My chest heaved up and down as I sat in my chair, unable to stop the water gushing from my eyes. I hiccupped from not being able to catch my breath. Soon my shirt was wet from all the tears and snot now dripping out of my nose. Dave sat across from me and silently watched.

"I'm sorry," I finally said after many minutes of this act.

"Don't be. You've got to let it out."

We sat in silence for a few more minutes before getting up to go to bed. There was nothing else that could be said to make the situation better.

We were all tense. Dave had his own versions of breakdowns, which looked more like fits of anger than anything else. He had experienced these moments throughout Emily's childhood, but they intensified now. He would rant angrily about not being able to just go out without finding a sitter or the overwhelming feeling of being trapped at the house. He would never be able to travel as much as he'd like or even enjoy a quick weekend away with his wife. *When do I get time alone with you? When will we stop watching cartoons? Would I ever be able to watch the news without interruption?* I would sit and listen to his rants, just like he would sit and watch me cry.

Among the breakdowns, though, we found ways to enjoy life. We went out to lunch when Emily was in school—those were our dates. Dave and I also continued our half-mile walks around the block. We went at least twice a day, and most days, three times. We got fresh air, talked with each other without interruption, and chatted with neighbors who were also out, while Sandy enjoyed the exercise she was getting coming along with us.

We were also getting closer to several friends in the neighborhood. They still didn't know all the intricacies of Emily's past, or even what we were currently going through, but they knew her (and our) limitations. They offered to babysit so Dave and I could go to that concert we really wanted to go to. They offered to take us out on their boat with no expectations of being out long. They'd say, "As soon as Emily is done, we'll turn around." On several occasions, our doorbell would ring and we would find a neighbor standing on our porch with a batch of homemade chocolate goodies they made for Emily. And our friends would offer to come hang out at our house, instead of going out, knowing it was just easier for us to not leave her. These moments, these types of friendships, got us through the long days.

≋ 23 ≋

Little Brothers

Ryan was also growing a bit moody during that time, probably a mix of hormones and our home life. Dave and I were stressed out, more than usual, and Emily, of course, still got most of the attention. Ryan didn't play with her anymore and had even outgrown the shows she watched on TV—she was stuck at seven years old, and now he was well past that. It was proving to be more and more of a struggle to do things together.

I decided to take the kids to visit Mike and Kim, who had recently moved to Minnesota, knowing we'd all get a little spoiled at their house. I tried to visit each of my brothers and their families with the kids every year, leaving Dave at home. It worked out well—the kids and I would get doted on by my family and Dave enjoyed the break from us. During this visit, we went to a beach that had a ramp for disabled people to use to enter the water. As Emily, Kim and I were lounging near the ramp, Ryan and Mike played Frisbee in the water. A gentleman who looked to be about 25 years old was gripping the bars of the ramp while standing in the water, watching. After a little while, he called to Mike in slow, thick speech, "Hey, guy, throw it here."

Mike looked his way and threw him the Frisbee. The man then gripped it with hands that didn't quite work and expertly threw it to Ryan. Ryan caught it and threw it to Mike, who then threw it to the new guy. This continued for a few minutes, and Mike yelled to the guy, "My name's Mike."

"Nice to meet you. I'm Doug," the man said slowly.

"Hey, Doug, I'm Ryan!" Ryan yelled over to him.

"Hey, Ryan," Doug said.

"Can you show me how you throw the Frisbee? That's cool," Ryan asked the man, who proceeded to show Ryan his grip.

The game continued for a while, and then it was time to go in. Mike commented later that night, after the kids went to bed, that he was impressed with Ryan's ease at the beach. He said it felt like he was there with a grown man, not a 10-year-old. To Ryan, it seemed, people with disabilities were no different than anyone else. He saw Emily and knew that she worked harder at most things, but that she also had feelings and a sense of humor and was able to do many, many things despite her disability. Ryan was wise beyond his years in the way he viewed and, more important, treated other people.

In the middle of Ryan's fifth grade year, I encouraged him to join the theater program Emily was in. They were going to do a take on *The Wizard of Oz*, and Alan, head of the program, always asked for Ryan to be a part of the show. I was hopeful it would help Ryan out of his funk and bring him and Emily a little closer.

He finally agreed, and a few months later, Dave and I beamed from the audience watching both of our kids confidently show their skills on that stage. Emily cackled and danced as a wicked witch, and Ryan, dressed as a scarecrow, wrangled a free-spirited boy a bit older than he was to his spot on the stage and cued him his lines. He laughed when his participant took over the microphone and ad libbed a song to which the audience cracked up. Ryan let him sing and then steered him back to his chair, accepting hugs from this boy all the while. This was all on stage in front of more than a hundred people, including his good friends and family in the audience. I swelled with pride at my loving son.

Shortly after the performance, the kids and I joined Dave on a work trip to Harrisburg, Pennsylvania. It was not far from Hershey Park, and we were excited to bring Emily to this chocolate mecca (Emily's obsession with chocolate never waned and she demanded it daily).

The first day we were there, we visited the park. It was a warm day, but nothing unusual, especially for us now having several North Carolina summers under our belts. We got on the first roller coaster we saw. I'm not a fan (and neither is Dave), but Emily, the daredevil, loved them and Ryan was anxious to try one. It didn't go especially fast or whip around too much, but when we got off, Emily looked sick. She said she didn't want to go on any other rides. Ryan, however, just had a taste of the thrill and wanted to continue. But it became clear that Emily was overheated and not recovering. We stopped in the air-conditioned gift shop, but that didn't seem to help either. Sadly, we were back in our hotel room before lunch.

We stayed in a one-bedroom suite that Dave usually had to himself on his business trips to that area. I joined Dave in the bedroom while the kids stayed in the living room—Emily on the pull-out sofa and Ryan on the floor, refusing to share the bed with Emily claiming he got kicked too many times during the last trip together. That night, Emily was asleep on the pull-out sofa by 7, so we dimmed the lights and turned down the TV. Ryan was flipping between cartoons and a baseball game, so Dave and I retreated to the bedroom to watch TV. At 8, though, I noticed the light went out in the kids' area and the TV turned off.

"What's going on, Ryan?" I asked, confused as to why he was turning everything off so early.

Annoyed, he remarked, "I might as well go to bed. I've been up since five o'clock this morning anyway with Emily."

The next day he proceeded to sulk because we went down to the hotel pool instead of back to the park. Finally, Dave whispered to me that maybe I should take him to Friendly's for an ice cream sundae and he would stay back at the hotel with Emily. Although I was totally perturbed by his sullen mood and didn't want to reward it, something needed to be done to salvage the trip. The ice cream outing just for him seemed to help. It was a reminder to us that although he didn't act out in obvious ways, Ryan was still young enough to be hurt by the limitations in our lives, especially on that vacation.

When we got home, we got word that the overnight camp of which we thought Emily aged out would allow Emily to come back for one more week that summer. That we were thrilled with this news was putting it mildly. We could all use a break. Not only would Emily love all the activities at camp, we thought it would be the perfect opportunity to take Ryan on a vacation with just us.

A month later, we dropped Emily off at her summer camp one last time and went to a beach resort with Ryan. I had no anxiety about leaving her there—she was so excited to go to camp I felt the excitement for her. And for five days Dave, Ryan and I were able to sit on the beach, eat at restaurants, go swimming in the pool, and stay out after the stars came out. Ryan could run on the beach and we could keep up, join him on the water slides and go through the lazy river together as a family. Except we weren't. A piece of our hearts was missing.

We kept that vacation secret from Emily. We felt guilty not including her on a trip to the beach and didn't know of a better way to address it, so we didn't talk about it.

"I feel like we live separate lives," I told Dave one evening after dinner.

"We do."

But the one-on-one time with Ryan proved to be time well spent. We enjoyed his company, and I think it gave him a boost of confidence. He did another performance with TOCS and announced that he wanted to shave his head for St. Baldrick's, a non-profit organization that raises money for childhood cancer research. They host events at various places where participants can sign up to raise money and then shave their heads in a show of support for cancer patients who lose their hair to chemotherapy.

I was taken aback by his announcement. He was now in middle school, and the stakes were high for looking different. I asked, "Are you sure you want to shave your head?"

"Yeah, of course."

"What are going to say if kids make fun of you?" I asked, trying to get him to think of the reality of shaving his head.

"Who's going to make fun of me for doing this? Besides, I'd just tell them I did it for kids with cancer." He made an excellent point. Maybe I was just going back to my insecure middle school days instead of seeing him for the confident boy he was.

He wrote an essay on why he wanted to do the fundraiser, a necessary step to take part in the event at his school. Then proceeded to go door to door, by himself, in our neighborhood to raise money. He collected a thousand dollars all on his own, far surpassing his goal of $200, and became one of the top fund raisers for his school. The following week, in front of his entire grade, he sat on the gym floor with just one other kid from his grade and had his head shaved. He was right. Everyone cheered and clapped while I sat in the audience with tears in my eyes, so proud of the young man he was becoming.

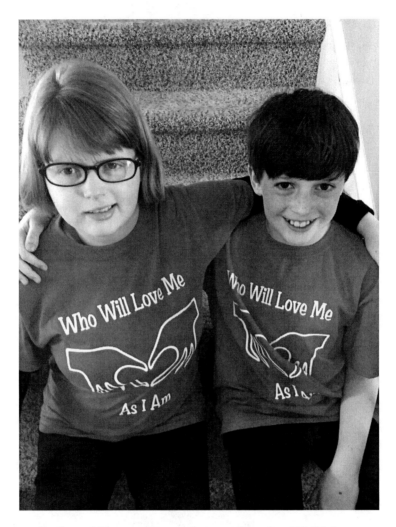

Emily and Ryan getting ready to perform in a TOCS show.

We knew life with a sister who had cognitive and physical disabilities wasn't easy. He always had to share his parents with her. Ryan never had both Dave and me at his sporting events; one of us was always home with Emily who didn't have the patience to sit through a game. But he also had a sister who continually drew him pictures that had hearts on them saying she loved him. He was still taken care of by her, much like he was when he was a newborn baby. She brought him a granola bar every morning when he woke up and liked making a spot on the couch comfy for him by spreading out a blanket. Most important, he learned that strength isn't from muscles but from watching his sister face challenge after challenge and never giving up. He learned grace by seeing her smile, every day, even though just getting dressed was difficult. The lessons learned from his big sister would get him through more in life than anything he would learn in school.

≋ 24 ≋

Blood Pressure

Miraculously, Emily's MRIs showed the tumor as stable despite stopping treatment. The chemotherapy, the few months she was on it, apparently did some work. The doctor suggested we move to having MRIs every six months unless she showed more symptoms. I was happy to have one less appointment to go to, as was Emily, for sure. I no longer felt the ups and downs of a looming MRI appointment. Emily's anxiety of going to the doctor's office was intensifying, and that's what I focused on when an MRI day was coming up instead of the MRI results themselves. We absolutely could not mention a doctor's appointment without Emily immediately tearing up, her lips trembling.

Emily started another summer break just as my job was growing more and more demanding. I would often get angry at myself for caring so much about my job and putting in the hours I did and Dave would continuously tell me to quit (and remind me that we moved to North Carolina so I wouldn't have to work). But Emily's routine was stressful in its own way. I couldn't take the endless repeated conversations and questions. I could recite every line of *SpongeBob* and *Lilo and Stitch*. I needed the time away from her, sitting at my desk in the next room, even if the time away was stressful.

Thankfully, at the height of my stress with work, the laws in North Carolina regarding the requirements around hiring aides, mainly using aides employed by state-approved agencies, changed. I was now allowed to hire my own aide and they were now allowed to drive participants places. This was years in the making, and I had been closely following its progress. The aides from state-approved agencies were typically not high quality. They got paid minimally because the agency took a cut of the Medicaid pay, which was not high to begin with. As the saying goes, you get what you pay for.

Finally, we could hire someone of our choosing. I started with an ad on a local Facebook page and got only one response, which didn't pan out. I then spread the word at Emily's school and with friends that we were looking to hire an aide for Emily. I was hearing crickets. I had three months to hire someone, and two months had already gone by with no one even interviewed yet.

The pressure was mounting, and my quest to find an aide for Emily was always on my mind. I was at our mailbox one afternoon chatting with our neighbor who was taking a walk with her granddaughter, Mia. Mia was Emily's age and had just graduated from high school but was planning on staying local for college.

That night, I thought, *Why not Mia?* She was only Emily's age, but maybe that would work out. I quickly got her number and asked if she would be interested in interviewing for the position. She responded, "Yes!"

We arranged a time for her to visit with me first, and I explained the position and expectations. I told her we were looking for someone to keep Emily actively engaged by playing with her, talking with her, going on walks, and so on. Mia was very articulate, had appropriate questions, and was overall an easy person to talk with—unlike many of the aides we had hired in the past. We arranged for Mia to stop by and hang out with Emily for a half hour or so. Emily had so much fun she didn't want to see Mia leave. We hired her on the spot.

From the get-go, Mia and Emily clicked. Mia talked to Emily like she would any of her friends. She suggested things to do, like crafts or playing the Wii. She joked with Emily, who joked right back. On Saturdays they went to the craft store for the kids' craft class. They would go out for McDonald's or stop at Dairy Queen for an ice cream. Emily was finally doing things that teenagers did with other teenagers. Mia didn't seem affected by the fact that she had to hold Emily's hand to balance her when she walked or that her memory escaped her most times. When Emily had a seizure, she just made sure she was sitting, without making a big deal of it, and then sat with her. I loved her.

Within a few months, the mood in our house eased. Emily now had someone to look forward to hanging out with. I didn't feel like I needed to monitor their relationship like I did with previous aides. I realized I could actually be productive during the time that Mia was with Emily. She came to the house in time to get Emily off the school cab and stayed until 5. This meant that I worked an entire day with barely any interruption. That hadn't happened in years.

My confidence in my ability to do my job soared. When Mia took Emily out on Saturdays, I hung out with Ryan. We played catch, went for walks, or ran errands—just the two of us. Beyond the practical reasons of having a few hours to ourselves each day, we loved that Emily finally had a friend again. It had been years since Emily had a special person in her life to have fun with, someone who wasn't her mom.

Mia would even babysit for us on weekend evenings. Dave and I now went out to eat at restaurants in Raleigh and attended concerts in addition to the parties in the neighborhood. Mia was the blessing to our family we didn't know we needed, and I finally understood my mom's insistence that having an aide would be beneficial.

We had yet another new routine now, and this one we were fond of. Both kids were in school and Mia hung out with Emily every day after school until 5. Dave was working his same job and going on the occasional business trip. I was still working full-time from home, going into the office for a meeting here or there. And Emily was healthy again—healthy for her. She still suffered from seizures, but her Crohn's disease was finally well managed, and the tumor was still remarkably stable. My mental breakdowns were happening less and less.

Dave was itching for a big trip. The sense of calmness in our house probably fueled his desire. We had already been on several family vacations over the last few years—visiting Jeff and his family, who now lived in New Mexico and visiting Mike and Kim, who recently moved to St. Louis, as well as a trip to visit Dave's grandma in Florida. Traveling had remained important to both Dave and me—even through all of Emily's hardships. Now, though, Dave was ready for a big, grown-up trip. He kept bringing it up, but with no overnight camp in which to leave Emily, he and I couldn't go on one together. After a few weeks of mumbling about traveling, he asked what I thought about him taking Ryan on a trip—just the two of them.

"I think that would be fantastic." I loved the idea that Ryan would get a chance to explore the world a bit. I was also thrilled with the idea because Dave would get the travel bug out of his system, and I could stay home with Emily. I couldn't stomach the stress involved with either bringing her or leaving her.

"Awesome. I was thinking of going to Iceland. I've been looking into it—there's some adventurous stuff we could do." He got out the iPad and showed me the tours available involving waterfalls, glaciers, and seeing the Northern Lights.

The plan was to go in the early spring when it was light enough during the day but dark at night so they could try to see the Northern Lights. The timing also coincided with Ryan's birthday. We talked with him about the idea of spending it in Iceland, and he thought that would be a fine way to spend his 13th birthday.

Once my mom learned of the trip, she offered to watch Emily so I could join them. "With Emily being in school and Mia there to help, I think we could manage."

Although grateful, I had to admit to my mom that it was just too stressful to coordinate everything involved in leaving Emily, and I'd be worried she might get sick or something might happen. Leaving her at camp, under the supervision of doctors, while I'm a few hours away is one thing. Leaving her at home while I leave the country is another. Besides, Dave was looking forward to some father-son time with Ryan. I was happy not to intrude on that.

A few weeks before their trip, Emily started complaining of headaches and neck pain. I grew concerned but didn't run to the doctor. Once I mentioned "doctor," lips would quiver and then she'd say she felt better. During the last several routine doctor appointments, in fact, she would tell the doctor as he or she was entering the room, "I'm fine. Can I go home now?"

On the Saturday before Easter she again complained of a headache. I gave her a Tylenol then suggested we go to Nana and Grandpa's house (which was always a treat for her). Within just a few minutes of getting there, Emily laid on their couch saying her neck hurt. Then she started crying. My mom looked at me like, *do something!*

"Do you think I should take her to Urgent Care?" I asked my mom.

"Yes," she said very rigidly. Like, *why haven't you taken her already?* This was also the same person who made me sit patiently for her Bridge game to end before taking me to the doctor to get my clearly broken arm set when I was just six years old.

So I took her to Urgent Care where we were told to take her straight to Duke's Emergency Room without going home. The doctor wasn't sure why she was having neck pain, but Emily's blood pressure was high enough to warrant an ER visit.

"Okay," was my resigned response. Although I wanted Emily to feel relief, I did not want to spend the rest of the day at Duke. Emily was upset. And I was hungry. My bad mood was settling in.

Within a half hour, quick by ER standards, we were sent back to a room in the Emergency Department, where a complete workup was ordered. A quick MRI showed that the shunt was working fine and there was no obvious tumor growth. She was then put on medicines to bring down her blood pressure and more doctors were consulted.

By 11 that night, still sitting in the little room in the Emergency Department, still hungry and now exhausted, I told the nurse we really needed to go home. Her blood pressure was elevated, but not nearly as high as it was when we arrived. Emily no longer had any head or neck pain and was growing frustrated at still being there. She had endured multiple pokes and an MRI while there (along with missing dinner), and it was way past when she liked to go to bed. In fact, when Emily asked me what time it was and I told her 11 o'clock, she exclaimed, "I'm missing lunch?!" To her, 11 o'clock only came one time a day, and that was lunchtime.

The nurse relayed my desire to go home to the doctor, who came to chat with me.

"I'd really like Emily to get admitted to figure out what's going on with her blood pressure. I've got some phone calls in with the nephrology department because I think she needs a kidney work-up done," the doctor gently explained to me, obviously not understanding my all-consuming goal to go home.

"Admitted? Her blood pressure is coming down. She feels fine now."

"I think it's best to admit her for more testing," she persisted.

"It's Easter tomorrow. What if we come in Monday for an

outpatient visit?" *Please let us go home, please let us go home, please let us go home.*

She paused, looking at me for a minute. "Let me put in another call to the department, and let's see if her blood pressure continues to drop. If it gets low enough, it'll probably be fine to go home."

I sat for the next 45 minutes staring at the blood pressure machine, willing the numbers to come down each time it took Emily's readings. Slowly but surely, they dropped below the threshold set by the ER doctor. We were out of there.

Emily happily went to sleep in her own bed that night and I did too, once I put together the Easter baskets. Dave whole-heartedly admits that if it weren't for me, the kids would have a sad, unfortunate childhood. They would get bags of candy handed to them instead of the artfully decorated baskets I put together year after year, which were strategically hid, along with the eggs decorated a few days prior, throughout the house.

The next morning, at Emily's usual wake-up time, we were awake, no matter she didn't go to sleep until almost 1 a.m. She waited until Ryan came downstairs closer to 7 before the two of them went off excitedly looking for the eggs and baskets. Ryan let her find the obvious ones while he hunted for the difficult ones, which weren't all that difficult to find. I put them wherever I could reach and the dog couldn't. That was about as thoughtful as I could get at 1 in the morning.

As we were getting ready to go to my parents' house for a big Easter brunch, my phone rang with a number I recognized coming from the hospital. It was a doctor from the Nephrology (Kidney) Department wanting us to come into the hospital for more testing and monitoring.

"Sure, when would you like us to come in?" I asked, impressed that they were calling on a holiday.

"Now. I'm not exactly sure why you were let go last night. She should have been admitted."

"Well, Emily was feeling better and her blood pressure was dropping with the medication. Plus, it's Easter today so I asked that we go home."

After going back and forth for a little bit, the doctor, getting sterner with each passing moment, got me to agree to bring her in that afternoon and told me to pack for a few days. I got off the phone with the doctor to find Dave loading the casserole dishes we were taking to brunch into the car. Ryan was already buckled in.

"That was the doctor. I need to bring Emily back in to get admitted."

"What? That's crazy. Can't you just bring her in tomorrow?" he asked.

"Apparently we shouldn't have been able to go home last night. He said she's too unstable to be home without monitoring."

He sighed audibly. "Well, what do you want to do?"

"I *want* to stay home with my family. I *want* to be able to work tomorrow. But I guess I need to take her to Duke." Now I was pissed. Like any of this was in my control.

He sighed again. "Can you at least have brunch with us and then go later this afternoon?"

"Fine. But he really wanted her in now. How about we take two cars to my parents and I just leave with Emily from there?"

"Fine," he relented, Emily's life controlling ours yet again.

I went in to quickly pack a bag for Emily and one for me. I was trying really hard not to let the anger I felt at the doctor, and now Dave, get to me. *Just get through brunch*, repeated in my head. We got to my parents' and let them know the plan while out of earshot from Emily. They knew we couldn't discuss any of this in front of her without making her cry. After an incredibly tense lunch with light, inane conversation, me upset about the whole situation, and Dave, now, upset over it too, we left for the hospital.

Once we were on the road, my mantra changed to *Just get through tonight*. We checked in at the Emergency Room and were escorted upstairs to an inpatient room fairly quickly. Emily's blood pressure was high, and she was put on a new medication to try to bring it down. She was also brought down for an ultrasound of her kidneys that afternoon. We met with a kidney specialist who explained the various tests he would be conducting to see if the kidneys might be causing the high blood pressure.

For Emily, being at the doctor's office was bad and sleeping at the doctor's was awful, but being put on a restrictive diet was pure torture. I learned that when we ordered her dinner that night from the hospital cafeteria that she was put on a no-salt diet. *Sorry, you can't have French fries. Nope, no macaroni and cheese, either.* It was a rough few days in the hospital. She was feeling better with her blood pressure under control with new medicines and she was bored with the stay. Every day, a new test was conducted that showed nothing wrong. Emily had some scarring on her kidney from the excessive UTIs as a child, but that was it. After three days, I was getting antsy as well. Dave and Ryan were leaving for Iceland at the end of the week and I absolutely wanted to be home before they left. I needed time with Ryan. I wanted to help him pack and do any last-minute shopping he might need. I wanted to hold him. He was leaving the country without me, and that, of course, caused a twinge of worry as it would with any mom.

On Wednesday, after many talks with the doctor about wanting to go home, we were able to go. Emily was put on a new blood pressure medicine the night before, and it finally dropped her pressure to the normal range. Emily survived the no-salt diet during her stay at the hospital and we had orders to continue watching her sodium levels at home. *Fine, anything! Just let us go home so I could hug my boys before they leave for a week*, was what went through my head.

Emily was tired when we got home. So tired she drifted in and out of sleep while sitting on the couch that afternoon. Dave kept saying, "She must be exhausted from the hospital stay—you never get good sleep there." I was slightly skeptical because she was full of energy—well, as much energy as Emily ever had, while we were at the hospital.

That afternoon, I helped Ryan get all his clothes together for the trip. We put piles of pants, shirts, socks and underwear on his desk so he was ready to pack on Friday. I pulled out his new winter coat and windbreaker and laid it on top of the piles. His hiking boots were sitting on the floor ready to go. Now, at least, if anything should come up again with Emily between now and Friday, at least he'd know what to pack. And I hugged him. I missed him already. It seemed he was growing and maturing so fast, especially compared to Emily. I knew my time with him was short. I hated being away from him. Unlike Emily, I knew he would someday leave our house and live his own life.

Ryan had gone to sleepaway camp the summer before for the first time and thrived in the environment. I knew he'd be fine on this trip with his dad. And that's what made me pause. Ryan was on the cusp of becoming a teenager and seemed so grown up. He could make himself snacks and light meals and do his own laundry (after nagging, of course). He was no longer the little boy so dependent on me—his growing-up years seemed to have raced by, especially compared to Emily's childhood, which has never ended. I spent so much time resentful that Emily would never "grow up," and here was my son, growing up too quickly. My heart and brain played a nasty game of tug of war—one begging him to stop maturing, the other making sure he grew up.

Emily went to bed at 7 that night, her usual time. And I was excited to sleep in my own bed again. At six in the morning, though, I heard Emily get up. It was an hour later than she usually got up. I quickly got up to see how she was feeling, and when I was halfway to her room, she called me in a panicked voice.

"Mom! My face! My face is tingling!" she cried.

She was sitting on her bed with her left hand covering her face, tears coming down her cheeks. I grabbed her and hugged her. "Your face is tingling? Does it hurt?"

"No, just tingling. It was scary."

"Oh, honey, I'm here. You're okay. Let me look." She dropped her hand, and I didn't see anything unusual.

"Let's go get you comfy on the couch," I said to her.

"My legs don't work," she said.

"What?!" I said as I helped her up, and she was right—she was dead weight. I stood behind her, looped my arms around her chest, and we shakily walked to the couch in the next room.

"What are you feeling right now? Is anything tingling or hurting? Do you have a headache?" I asked, concerned she just had a stroke.

"I'm okay now."

I looked at her for several minutes. She always had a right-side weakness which resulted in the right side of her face drooping—one of the signs of a stroke. How could I tell if she actually had one?

"My forehead is a little tingly again," she said.

This time I saw a lump on her forehead, above her left eye.

"My lips are tingly now."

I stared at her face for another few minutes.

"It went away, it's fine now," she said after a minute.

She was calm, and I was trying to be. I turned on the TV for her and went to wake up Dave. He came downstairs after I explained what was going on with Emily. The absolute *last* thing I wanted was to go back to the hospital, and I wanted reassurance from someone that I didn't need to take her. Dave would tell me I didn't need to; I was sure of it.

"How are you feeling, Em?" Dave asked.

She lazily looked at him and slurred, "Fine," then went back to watching TV.

"She had a stroke," he said to me. *Shit. Shit. Shit.*

"Do I take her in? What would they actually do for her?" I asked. Pleaded. "Maybe I just call the kidney doctor and let them know."

"Yeah—call them and see what they say," he said.

I found our discharge papers with the number to call for various reasons, none of which were face tingling and inability to walk, and dialed the number. I talked with the on-call doctor who thought the tingling, especially around her lips, sounded like an allergic reaction to the new blood pressure medicine. She said to take her off the medicine, and she'd prescribe a new medication for her to take instead.

"But what about her not being able to walk?" I asked.

"I'm not sure what that's about. But try the new medicine and let us know if she shows any more symptoms. And make sure to bring her in for her follow-up appointment next week." I stopped the conversation and didn't pursue it any longer. I wanted—no, *needed*—to believe that the only thing that occurred was an allergic reaction.

I relayed to Dave the conversation. I'm not sure if it was wishful thinking, the power of denial or pure hope that made us go along with this diagnosis of allergic reaction. Deep down, I felt that she had a stroke. I also knew there was nothing that could be done for it. Emily promptly fell asleep on the couch. We lifted her legs up, rotated her around, put a blanket on her, and let her sleep.

⇛ 25 ⇚

Iceland

I obviously had Emily stay home from school that day, even though she had already missed the first half of the week being in the hospital, and the week prior she was home on spring break. She kept saying she felt fine and wanted to go to school. She missed her teachers and friends. But she slept on and off for most of the day, and she started drooling a bit. She hadn't done that before. We would just hand her a tissue, and she would wipe the spit from her chin and go on with whatever it was she was doing. Her legs started working again, but her balance was off. We held her hand anytime she needed to go somewhere. Something had happened inside her brain.

I was thankful that Dave and Ryan were leaving for their trip in two days. I knew the week would be rough with her, and having Dave witness it would cause him stress. I didn't want to feel his anxiety when I had my own to deal with. On Friday morning, I fed Emily breakfast and she announced she wanted to go to school. I thought, *Why not?* The school was two miles from the house and her teacher would let me know if she needed to come home. Plus, I could spend the day uninterrupted with Ryan, who didn't have school that day. I got Emily in the cab and texted her teacher that she was on her way in and needed help walking. I had been emailing her updates all week, so she knew what had been going on up until that point.

At 10:30, I got the text to pick her up. She was sleepy and drooling. The teacher also said that she made her use a wheelchair, and Emily was quite upset about needing to use it. So Emily came home to sit on the couch while Dave and Ryan prepared to leave the next day for Iceland. Dave and I hadn't discussed her health since the

221

phone call with the on-call doctor the day prior. As he was getting his suitcase ready, he asked, "Are you sure you're going to be okay?"

"Yes! I'll be fine. She's good—just sleepy," I replied. And I meant it. I was confident that with a few more days of lying low, she'd recover.

The next morning, I hugged my son and told him to have a blast. I kissed Dave good-bye and told him to take care of my little boy. With a big lump in my throat, I watched them drive up the street and head to the airport. I walked back into the house and proceeded to clean every inch of the house as a way to use up my nervous energy. Emily did her usual amount of drawing pictures but spent the remainder of the day watching TV or nodding off on the couch. By 6:30 she wanted to go to bed and I let her.

It was now my turn to lie on the couch. The house was eerily silent. It was a very new feeling to have no one home except Emily— and have her be sleeping in her room. I thought I would be giddy to have everything to myself. Instead, I just covered myself up with a blanket and called the dog up to the couch to join me. I watched reality shows on Bravo, finally having the remote to myself with no one to judge my selection of shows, and was asleep by eight o'clock.

The next morning, I got a phone call from Dave which put me over the moon. He and Ryan made it safely to Iceland, and they'd already been out exploring, having a great time. Their happiness and excitement bubbled over to me and infused me with renewed energy. I showed Emily the pictures they'd sent, all bundled up, enduring the cold wind of the area, and Emily said, "I'm glad I'm not there!" We told Emily that they were going on a trip, knowing she wouldn't like the cold weather, and as predicted, she was relieved to not have to go.

Emily tried going to school again on Monday, but I received the text to pick her up by noon. Well, progress, I thought. Her teacher had relayed the same thing—she just wants to sleep. And she was still upset that she had to use a wheelchair at school. She came home and napped on the couch for a few hours. At that point, I was just happy to have the time to work. I had an extremely busy week planned with a very important meeting in a few days that I wanted to prepare for.

Dave and Ryan were sending me texts, and I got to speak to them each morning they were gone. They were having an adventure of a lifetime and I was thrilled for them both. Dave kept asking how Emily was doing and I said, "Better and better!" But reality was soaking in for me. She was not the same. She was still very tired, and her coordination was abysmal. I had to get her undressed in the evenings because she could no longer take her clothes off like she used to. I had to brush her teeth for her instead of just put the toothpaste on the toothbrush for her to do it herself. Watching her walk her usual path from her bedroom to the kitchen was like watching a pinball getting shot through an arcade game. She bounced back and forth from the couch to the wall, finally making it to the kitchen, where she would hold on to the counters to steady herself as she walked.

On Wednesday morning, the day of my important meeting in the office, I sent Emily off to school again. She'd been making it at least a few hours each day and I kept hoping that it would be no different that day. *Just make it until noon,* was my morning mantra. Instead, I got the text at 8:30 that she wanted to go home to sleep. *Dammit!* I quickly called my mom and asked if she and my dad could watch her while I went to my meeting.

I finished getting dressed, quickly picked Emily up from school, and dropped her off at my parents' house—using all my might to walk her up the stairs and plop her on their couch. I didn't have time to spare, so I just yelled, "She's tired and needs a hand to hold onto in order to walk. Thanks—be back in a few hours!"

I got to my meeting on time and rushed through it, even though I had spent hours preparing for it and wanted to be thoughtful and thorough. Even so, my presentation was well received. But instead of staying to schmooze with the executives around the table after the meeting like my colleagues, I rushed over to my parents' house. I had to quickly turn off my thoughts regarding work and get Emily. I could think about work again once we were settled back at home.

Once home, I got Emily settled on our couch, where she promptly fell asleep. Only now could I get back to work. I was frustrated—no, angry—with the situation. I left work, letting my colleagues get the face-to-face time with executives, while I went back to a computer 10 miles away in my home. I kept comforting myself with the knowledge that the only way I *could* hold a job was by doing it from home. And I reminded myself that I wasn't in it to climb that corporate ladder anyway. A feeling of sadness and disappointment in myself that I was angry about work, pushing aside my worry for Emily, crept over me.

I thought about my flexible work schedule again the next day as I took Emily back to the hospital for her scheduled follow-up appointment with the kidney specialist. He walked into the room and asked how she was doing now that she was off the medication that supposedly caused a reaction. I explained the sleepiness and lack of coordination. He looked concerned and conducted a baseline exam of her.

"This looks like a neurological problem."

"Well, that's what I thought, too," I admitted with dread.

"I'm going to see if her neurologist is in clinic right now. Hold on." He left the room, and Emily leaned her head against my shoulder and fell asleep. Fifteen minutes later, he came back saying he couldn't find him, but the nurse was working on tracking him down.

It was Ryan's birthday. He was officially a teenager. The night before, he video chatted with me as he stood outside their cabin watching the Northern Lights and shared his view with me. It was amazing to see, even if it was on a little phone screen. At least, I thought, if the neurologist wants to do further testing or admit Emily to the hospital, Ryan's birthday wouldn't be ruined. They were having another fun day in Iceland, which made my heart happy, even though I longed to be there with them celebrating Ryan's birthday together.

The nurse finally came back in the room but just to let me know that Emily's neurologist was out of town. He was expected back later that night and would be in contact with me. We could go home since it was more pressing to see the neurologist, the kidney specialist confident that her kidneys were stable. I stood Emily up, using both hands to balance and right her. The nurse followed us out of the room and asked if she'd like a wheelchair. Emily quickly said, "No."

"It's okay, I've got her." Emily was my height but lighter than me. I knew exactly how to hold and balance her. I swung my purse over my left shoulder like I've been doing for 17 years, since Emily learned to walk, and took her left hand in my right hand. Off we walked, slowly down the hallway toward the parking lot.

Dave and Ryan were coming home the next day. Emily was only slightly better than when Dave left her a week earlier. She still needed a hand to hold onto in order to walk. I still had to brush her teeth for her and get her completely dressed and undressed. And she was still really tired. I was well rested, though. Instead of the girls' nights and binge-watching I was planning while the boys were away, I went to bed early. Extremely early. Most nights I was asleep by 8:30.

When I heard the garage door open on Friday, I ran outside and waited for Ryan to get out of the car. I gave him a big hug and asked how it was. "Great! And I'm 13 years old now," he grinned as he handed me his cell phone. We had a deal that he could get on certain social media once he was a teenager. He hadn't forgotten. I typed in the password, and he downloaded the apps he wanted and ran into the house. Dave had grabbed luggage out of the truck and gave me a kiss.

"How are you doing?" I asked.

"Good. It was a great trip."

I was relieved to hear that he had fun too.

"How's Em?" Dave asked as we walked into the house.

"Good. Well, the same. The neurologist called, and we have an appointment set up to see him early next week. We'll see what he says."

We changed gears back to him and Ryan, though. I wanted to hear all about the trip. And I needed the distraction. An hour later my parents and Jeff, in town for work, came over bearing take-out. We all sat around the TV, which Dave had hooked up to his phone, and watched a slideshow of their trip to Iceland. For the next hour I lived vicariously through Ryan and Dave excitedly sharing stories of their adventure. Emily sat on the couch watching, drool hanging from her lip, and half asleep. She went to bed as soon as the slideshow was over.

I was excited to finally meet with the neurologist a few days later. After examining her and listening to what had happened, the neurologist shrugged and said, "Radiation vasculopathy" to the intern also in the room. I continued with my own diagnosis: "I think she had a stroke."

"I'm not sure," the neurologist said. "This could just be an effect from the radiation treatment she endured years ago, but I'll set you up with my colleague who specializes in strokes because this is not due to her epilepsy. When one has a seizure, the symptoms last for the length of the seizure and then stop. Emily clearly has something else going on causing the fatigue and lack of coordination." He said to the intern, "Get her scheduled for an MRI and MRA of her brain and neck. I want it done quickly, as soon as possible, within the week."

Now I was looking forward to another doctor appointment to get some answers. The MRI and angiogram of Emily's brain and neck would surely show something. The next day, Emily went back to school, finally making it through a full day. I worked like I always did, juggling my days between doctor appointments and meetings.

When Emily had been in the hospital for nine days recovering from HSP, I let my boss know a very brief version of what was going on. I had to tell him because I could not accept any meeting requests during that time—if Emily had a pain attack, she screamed and needed my attention. My supervisor accepted the information with the human reaction "I'm sorry to hear that. Just do what you need to do." I worked very independently with minimal support, and my supervisor worked the same way—he was just as overworked as I was and had no one to cover for me if I wasn't available. God, I missed my old job where my supervisor's reaction was always "Take all the time you need."

Now, with the number of doctor appointments ramping up, including MRIs which were at least half-day events, I felt I needed to let my boss know what was going on. I happened to be in the office for another meeting with my supervisor. As we wrapped up the meeting, he asked if I had any other updates.

"Yes. I just wanted to let you know that I've been working funky hours lately because my daughter has had numerous doctor appointments. It looks like she'll have several more over the upcoming weeks. I'll take time off when I need to, otherwise I work early and late to make up for lost time."

"What's going on?" my boss asked.

"We think she had a small stroke but we're trying to get to the bottom of it," I flatly replied. I was in professional Amy mode.

"Oh, wow. I hope everything goes okay. Is there anything you need?"

"Just your continued flexibility with my schedule. I really appreciate that," I remarked. I long ago lost the hope of making meaningful friendships at this job like I had at my other places of employment.

"Of course. No problem."

And then it was back to business. The company had been going through numerous reorganizations and layoffs over the last year, and everyone seemed on edge and overworked. It didn't matter that Emily may have had a stroke—when I was in front of my computer, I had to somehow forget the stress of home. As ludicrous as it was, though, I appreciated that I had something else to concentrate on and think about.

Two more days went by, and I hadn't received a call about when the MRI and angiogram would be. I called the neurology clinic and left an urgent voicemail for the nurse saying I needed to know when it was scheduled—the doctor said he wanted it done that week. In my heart of hearts, I knew Emily had a stroke. There was nothing that could be done about it medically, so I wasn't sure why I so badly needed the doctor to confirm this, but I did. Perhaps I just needed validation that yes, something major occurred which had made Emily unable to walk independently or do other tasks she used to do. I needed to understand this step backward.

Another day went by before the nurse called me back. That poor nurse. She told me that the MRI and angiograms hadn't been scheduled yet, but it probably wouldn't be until next month. With this news, I became unhinged. "Are you kidding me? They haven't been scheduled yet, and it will be a month before she probably has the scans? The doctor said he wanted it done immediately!"

"I'm sorry. She'll need to have anesthesia for this one because it's of the head and neck, and the angiogram makes it longer as well. The coordination needed among departments makes it a little more difficult to schedule."

"No. The doctor said he wanted it done this week." I was shaking and couldn't stop the tears from pooling in my eyes.

"I don't see any rush orders with this," she calmly told me.

"Then the intern who was placing the orders didn't do it properly. I'm telling you he wanted it done this week!" I heard my voice getting louder and louder, tears now dripping down my face.

"I can talk with him, but, honestly, I don't think it will happen this week—anesthesia has been booked."

"My daughter had a stroke and I can't get a fucking MRI scheduled?!" I lost it. I was bawling and yelling at this poor nurse. I still didn't understand why it was so important to me that Emily have this scan—it would change nothing. I realized all of that after I yelled at her, along with the realization that I was losing myself. Who was this ugly person, screaming and swearing?

"I'm sorry. I'm sorry I yelled at you," I said to her, in between sobs.

"It's okay. It's really okay. I'm sorry you're going through this," the nurse said.

During a minute of silence, I pulled myself together. "Thank you for understanding. I'm so sorry I yelled at you." I finally calmed down and stopped crying.

"It's okay. I'll call you back once everything is scheduled."

"I heard yelling. What happened?" Dave asked, walking downstairs to where I was standing.

I told him about my conversation with the nurse. He didn't say anything. It was just another moment for me, for us. Six months earlier, I had battled the insurance company over a new prescription for Emily's Crohn's disease. Much like today, it had ended with me angrily yelling and swearing at an insurance representative. I hung up the phone on the rep, made myself a gin and tonic, even though it was only three o'clock in the afternoon on a Wednesday, and sat on my front porch, stewing. Dave came outside and asked if I was okay and why there was a lime in my water. I told him everything, including the screaming match with the insurance representative, and that it really wasn't water.

"Those poor insurance reps have no idea who they're up against. You'll get it figured out," he calmly told me.

Dave was right. Within the week, I got the go-ahead to use the specialty pharmacy I needed to use.

The nurse called me back the next day. She hesitantly, and apologetically, told me that while they could schedule the images of Emily's brain, the insurance company denied the angiogram of her neck. She told me the doctor was working on resubmitting the letter to the insurance company, further explaining the need for the procedure.

I'm sure the nurse just wanted to be done with my case and thought I could lose my mind again at any given moment. She was probably right, but I knew that she wasn't the one deserving of my anger—the insurance company was. And, for some reason, I resigned my typical fight mode. I just didn't have it in me anymore. Almost 20 years of battling insurance companies was enough. They won.

"Really? Did they say why they're not approving it?" I genuinely, calmly asked the nurse.

"Just that they didn't deem it necessary. It's maddening because the case notes clearly state that she's been experiencing neck pain leading up to the event," the nurse responded.

"Well, hopefully the letter from the doctor will fix it." And that was it. The nurse concluded the call after giving me the date of the MRI and angiogram of Emily's brain. I didn't call my insurance company to rip them a new one like I would have typically done. I just let it be and went back to my computer in work mode, thoughts of Emily, the nurse, and the insurance company turned off.

We met with the neurologist who specialized in strokes, and while she thought Emily's symptoms certainly sounded like a stroke, she was also concerned that an autoimmune issue might be causing some of the symptoms. She told me she would call after Emily's MRI and angiogram of the brain and set up a follow-up appointment.

The following week, after bringing a tearful Emily to yet another MRI appointment with pokes, the doctor called me with the results. There was indeed a sign of a stroke on the angiogram, but it could have been the one she had when she was seven years old. There were also some abnormalities with the arteries in her brain, but with no baseline angiogram to compare them to, it was hard to determine what abnormalities were new. The neurologist ended the conversation by telling me that she would continue to bring Emily's case up at various department meetings and get more eyes on the films.

Things were back to routine, a new routine. I got Emily completely dressed and undressed each day, brushed her teeth, and helped her walk. When she was in school, she used a wheelchair, and we received almost daily text messages from the teacher stating Emily was napping, had a seizure, or was ticked about needing to use the wheelchair. Her drooling never quite went away, especially when she was tired. Emily had taken a break from the theater program she had been in for so long, saying, "I don't want to do it. I will be too tired." She spent her free time drawing pictures or watching TV. Thanks to YouTube and Netflix, we added some of her old favorites that she loved to the mix—*Dragon Tales, Clifford,* and *Arthur.*

She watched these shows on a loop, as these were the only ones that she had interest in and could follow. Mia still came over regularly and noticed the decline, stating Emily got tired very easily and had to really be coaxed into doing some activities. I was tied to my computer working anytime I wasn't helping Emily. Ryan was back in school for his last quarter of middle school. And Dave continued to work and sometimes travel. Our outings dwindled, but we did make it to some neighborhood gatherings.

Despite her setbacks, Emily continued to start each day with a smile, a hug for me, and a good mood. The pictures she drew were of flowers, hearts, and rainbows. The only signs of frustration she showed with the new situation was embarrassment of her drooling and of needing to use a wheelchair at school. Her teacher would sometimes text me to say that Emily was having a rough day. But Emily would get out of the cab every single day and say, "My day was great!" Dave would ask Emily how her day was every night at dinner, and she'd answer, "Awesome sauce." Always. And I would smile at her, loving the outlook, wishing and hoping it would rub off on me.

Emily continued to argue with her teacher about the need for a wheelchair. "I walk fine," she would tell her teacher. "Just have someone hold my hand," she would counter if the teacher said she felt safer with her in a chair. At home, she would complain to me about using the wheelchair in school. "What exactly do you not like about using the wheelchair?" I finally asked, tired of this daily fight.

"I don't want to be stuck in it," Emily said, her lips trembling.

"What do you mean, stuck?"

"I don't want to be stuck in it. I know how to walk."

Oh. Oh, my sweet girl. She was afraid of being wheelchair bound. How did I not realize that *she* was worried about losing her abilities? I hugged her and told her that I knew she could walk and that wasn't going away. *Please don't let her completely lose the ability to walk*, I added to my growing list of prayers.

I tried explaining that she only needed to use the wheelchair when it was the safer alternative and that she could walk if it was safe. (I knew the teacher only had Emily use one to move through the hallways and for her gym class). She sighed at me and, with a roll of her eyes, said, "Fine." The next morning, I found a note in her school bag that Emily had written to her teacher. It read, "My mom says I don't need to use the wheelchair." I kept the note in there and texted the teacher our actual conversation, then wished her luck.

Dave and I took more and more walks around the block and did a lot more talking about Emily's health. Emily hadn't rebounded, even after several months. It was hard to figure out what the future would look like. Our daily life was harder than it was before—I couldn't run to the store with Emily anymore, even just to pick up one thing. It was difficult to balance her while holding an item and then pay for it. We found it more challenging to bring her out in general, even just to neighbors' houses. So we stayed home more and more. We noted that it was interesting that we no longer stressed about the tumor growing—instead, we worried about all these other systems that seemed to be failing her.

I gradually turned into a wreck. There were various weekly doctor appointments, prescription pick-ups and refills at a rapid rate, Emily needed constant assistance, and now she was out of school for the summer. Meanwhile, my job grew even more demanding with layoffs occurring at a regular rate. My mood was tense. Instead of relaxing on the couch after Emily went to bed, I worked. I logged into work when I woke up at 6 for the day, often meeting and instant messaging with my colleagues in Europe before the sun was up. Dave was trying to be supportive by letting me know, on numerous occasions, that I didn't need to be working. But I was adamant. I liked the distraction work was from my home life. I was in control of my work. It was the one thing in my life I *could* control. I was good at it and I liked the paycheck. I didn't worry as much about Ryan going off to college in a few years or taking care of Emily for the rest of our lives with my salary fattening up our savings account.

The summer ended, and we realized we never made it to the beach, one of Emily's (and my) favorite places. I searched house rentals online and found a handicapped accessible home—one-floor living, right on the beach, at the Outer Banks. There was a week available in October. Perfect. The secret that North Carolina natives are privy to is that fall is the best time to go to the beach. The water is still warm from the summer, and the weather is exceptional. Plus, no tourist crowds!

I was really looking forward to our week away. I couldn't wait for Emily to see the beach every day that we were there. I was anticipating Ryan spending his days in the water, riding the waves. I envisioned Dave and me sitting on the deck, snacking on cheese and crackers, drinking a cocktail, and watching the ocean crash onto the beach. We were even bringing the dog. Sandy would love the water. I blocked my calendar at work and took vacation days so that I would not feel obligated to check my messages.

The day before we left, Emily's teacher let me know that Emily had a rough day. She was very tired, and the drooling was bad, frustrating her. As I relayed this to Dave, I added, "Good thing we leave for the beach tomorrow!"

"She's been so tired. This will be great for her," he agreed.

≈ 26 ≋

The Beach

The next morning, I walked downstairs at 6:30 after deciding to sleep in a little on my first vacation day of the week. Emily was sitting at her usual spot on the couch watching TV, like I found her most every morning. She didn't make any motion to get up, like she usually did, though, when I entered the room.

"Hi, Em. You excited for the beach today?" I asked.

"Mmhmm," she nodded.

Then I noticed that she was drooling. A lot. Like a faucet turned on in her mouth. "Are you all right?"

"Uh-huh."

"Do you feel tingly anywhere?"

"No," she said with a smile now.

She looked out of it, and the drool wasn't stopping. I handed her a washcloth to wipe the spit hanging from her chin. About 45 minutes later Dave came downstairs, looked at Emily, then looked at me with wide eyes.

"She hasn't moved from the couch and the drool is out of control."

"Uh, yeah. She's completely out of it."

I sighed audibly. Then Dave did. "What do you want to do about the beach? Should we still go?" I asked him.

"Well, we can sit on the couch here or we can sit on the couch at the beach. I choose the beach," he said.

I paused only slightly before agreeing with him. These were the decisions we had to make. Do we give up or do we continue on?

I brought Emily some food to pick at on the couch, which she did. Then I stood her up. As I expected, she had a lot more trouble

233

walking now than before. I wasn't sure how she made it from her bedroom to the couch unless today's stroke, or whatever it was, happened after she was on the couch. After taking her to the bathroom, I sat her in the car and buckled her seatbelt.

Ryan was already seated and was very quiet. I handed Emily a towel to use to dab her mouth and laid another one across her chest to act like a bib. She just smiled at me. Then Sandy jumped in the car and stood on top of Ryan, making him wince in pain and then laugh, easing the tension in the car. I shut the door, grabbed the rest of my things, and got settled in the front seat. Dave locked up the house, jumped in the driver's seat, and we took off for the beach.

Emily still hadn't said much, really anything at all, during the car ride. Her drooling was constant. I kept turning around to look at her and she was gazing out the window. When we stopped at McDonald's for lunch, Dave stayed in the car with Emily and the dog. As Ryan and I walked in to get the food, he asked, "What's wrong with Emily?"

"We're not sure, but she may have had a small stroke," I answered, trying to be honest yet not cause panic.

"Is that why she's drooling?"

"It could be. A stroke is when blood doesn't get to an area of the brain, and that area stops working. She's not in pain, though, and she'll be all right," I said, reassuring him and myself. Ryan remained silent. "She's going to be okay," I said.

"I know," he said. At 13, though, this was his response to most things.

We brought the food back to the car, and as I was questioning why we thought it was a good idea to bring the dog, I put a napkin on Emily's lap and handed her French fries. She painstakingly slowly ate one fry. I opened the box of chicken nuggets and put those down next to the fries. Ten minutes later, after she had eaten two nuggets, I handed her a cup of ice water with a straw. As I held the cup, she tried drinking. She stopped and told me, "It's not working."

I lifted the straw out of the cup and couldn't find a defect. I jumbled the ice around in the cup and said, "Here, try again."

I watched as she sucked with all her might, and the water went halfway up the straw then stopped. I then tried the straw and effortlessly got a sip of water. She tried again and I made eye contact with Dave and shook my head.

Dave just put his head down.

I took the lid off the cup and lifted it to her lips, and she could finally take some sips of water. After she ate one more French fry, I asked if she had enough to eat and drink. Yes, she nodded. So I packed up everything and got settled back into the car for the rest of the drive to the beach.

"Do you think I need to call the doctor? She can't even suck water through the straw." I whispered to Dave.

"Well, yes, at some point. What do you think they'll do?" he asked.

"Nothing. More images and tests. It can all wait. I just want her, and us, to enjoy the beach." I hated that I struggled with whether to take Emily to the doctor. If this was someone who hadn't had medical issues all her life, it was a no-brainer to take her to the doctor. But this wasn't anyone ordinary. This was Emily. She had suffered from so much already. A few days of denial on the beach seemed like a good call.

"Then wait until we get home. Let's enjoy this trip. God knows how many others she'll be able to go on." And that was the hard truth. We both had the unsettling feeling that we didn't know how much longer she would be with us or if this was the last time she would go to the beach.

The beach house was everything it promised to be online. We were able to walk Emily into the house and sit her at the kitchen table while we unloaded and unpacked our things. I moved her to the deck overlooking the ocean while we explored the house and picked bedrooms. One of the rooms had two twin beds, and we decided it was best for me to sleep with Emily in that room. I would worry about her otherwise.

Emily seemed to have "woken up" a bit as we settled into the house. She chatted a little, saying, "I like this house. I like the beach." Not long after dinner, she asked to go to bed, and we obliged. Her eyes were closed by the time I got the covers up to her chin. We left the bedroom door open, and Dave taught Ryan how to play pool in the rec room. I happily joined them in a few games and enjoyed the denial that swept over us that night.

Emily slept all night, not waking until 5:30 the next morning. I walked her to the couch and found *SpongeBob* playing on TV, then brewed my pot of coffee. She was contentedly watching TV, so I brought the dog out and sat on the deck to watch the sun rise over the ocean. I had done this on numerous vacations with Emily. I learned to revel in the seemingly wicked hour she awoke by watching the sun rise, magically turning the scene from dark to light. I sat with my mug of coffee, alone with the dog. I thought of all the things Emily had endured in her short 19 years. How much she had suffered. And yet she was so happy. She continued to smile and tell us how much she loved all of us, day in and day out. It was that thought that stopped me from feeling sorry for myself. If Emily could enjoy these moments, we should too.

That morning, we trudged all our beach crap out to the sand. Then we brought Emily and sat her in a chair on the sand. Within 20 minutes, she was overheated—bright red and saying, "I'm hot," even though it was not quite 80 degrees. Dave took her back to the house, and I stayed with Ryan as he ran in and out of the ocean. We then walked with the dog down the beach, which we had to ourselves, other than the crabs running away from us. Ryan and I finally meandered back to the house where Emily dozed on the couch, and I broke my promise to leave work behind and checked my messages. I ended up working for an hour, mostly to distract myself from the dark thoughts that were starting to percolate in my brain.

In the afternoon we went to the Wright Brothers Memorial, where I discovered that Emily, truly, could barely walk. I could get her to take about 20 steps and that was it. It was too much of a struggle to get her to keep walking. So Dave took Ryan to various areas of the park, and Emily and I stood like statues on the sidewalk watching them. There was a bench not even 10 feet from where we were, but it seemed like a mile away. A park ranger walked by and asked if we needed a wheelchair or assistance. I said no, as if on autopilot to deny help. Instead, we waited in that spot until Dave came back with Ryan and unlocked Emily from my side.

My denial of the graveness of the situation was fading away. We went back to the car and drove to another area of the park. I screamed at Dave that we needed to go home, something was wrong

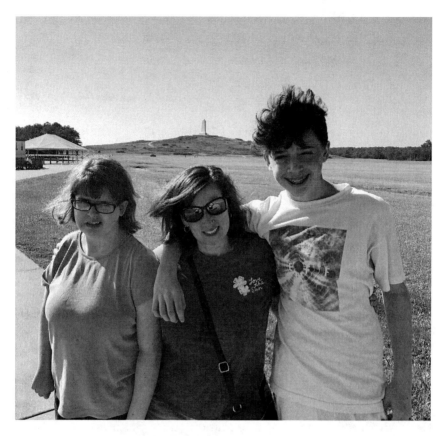

Emily, me and Ryan at the Wright Brothers National Memorial in the Outer Banks of North Carolina.

with Emily, but he just parked the car and said, "Why don't you and Ryan hike that trail to check out what's up there? I'll stay here with Emily."

I stared at him blankly, and Ryan jumped out of the car. The screaming must have been in my head. I swallowed back the sob that wanted to come out and got out of the car. I put on a smile, suddenly remembering that I needed to enjoy these moments that I had with Ryan, and we hiked to the top of the monument. We stood next to each other, Ryan at 13 years old already looming six inches over me, and we took in the view of the Outer Banks.

When we got back to the beach house that afternoon, after talking with Dave, I stood on the deck and finally called the neurologist who specialized in strokes and explained everything that had happened. She repeated everything back to me and summed up Emily's current state by saying, "She's lost her sparkle."

"Yes. Yes, that's exactly it. She's lost her sparkle."

And that's what scared me the most. I could deal with her not walking. I could deal with the drool. But, please, don't dampen her spirit.

"Do you need help with her? Do you want me to admit her to a hospital near you at the shore?" the doctor asked me.

"No, we've got her and can care for her. That's not necessary."

"Are you sure? I can easily get her admitted because I know it's got to be hard."

"I'm sure but thank you," I said firmly though I truly appreciated that she recognized that we were in a difficult situation. At that moment, no one else understood. I hadn't called my mom or my brothers. I hadn't told anyone. It was me, Dave, Ryan, and this doctor.

"I'm sorry to do this, but I do need her to have a scan, and it needs to be as soon as possible. You'll need to cut your vacation short." She said exactly what I was expecting to hear.

"I know. It's okay. We'll come home."

"All right, I'll call you back shortly once it gets scheduled. And call me if you change your mind about admitting her."

As promised, she called me back five minutes later with instructions for Emily's scan that was scheduled for Saturday morning. I told Dave, and he was expecting the news as well. I thought he might get angry about cutting our vacation short, but he didn't. In fact, a look of relief washed over him when I relayed that the doctor was going to see her that weekend. That night, while we played pool with Ryan, we let him know that we had to leave the next day in order for Emily to go to the doctor.

"Okay. That's fine," he said with a smile and a nod. Ryan no longer seemed to get upset with us when plans went sideways. Thank God he turned into an easy, understanding guy and didn't make this difficult situation even more difficult.

The next morning, Dave suggested we do something adventurous with Ryan before we left.

"Why don't we rent jet skis—you and he can go, and I'll sit with Emily. Take her for an ice cream or something," Dave suggested to me.

"I don't want to jet ski. But you can take him, and I'll sit with Emily."

"Why don't you want to jet ski?" Dave asked.

"Because I'm a total wimp these days. I'll go as fast as a turtle, and it won't be fun for him. I'll take him kayaking, though, if he wants to do that." I truly hated the grown-up I was becoming.

"Ryan," Dave called over to him in the next room, "we're thinking of jet skiing or kayaking this morning. Which would you prefer?"

"Jet skiing!" was his answer, of course.

Emily and I watched Dave and Ryan jet off in the sound before driving off to find an ice cream parlor. We quickly found one, and I struggled to get her up the six steps to the entrance. I plopped Emily down in the first seat we came across, my arms shaking from the effort to get her up the stairs, and ordered her a cup of chocolate ice cream. I sat across from her and held her bowl still, while she slowly spooned the gooey goodness into her mouth. I wiped her mouth after each bite but then gave up; she was just going to be a mess.

There was only one other couple in the place, and I noticed the woman went to the claw arcade game in the corner. When she captured a stuffed animal, she whooped a "Yes!" and did a happy dance, giggling all the while. She then promptly walked over to our table and placed it next to Emily.

"For you!" the woman announced.

Emily grinned a big chocolate smile. "Thank you!" She was genuinely smitten, as was I.

"Thank you! That's so sweet," I told the woman. She just grinned and walked back to her table. I wasn't surprised at this gesture. It happened regularly. Emily's spirit had a way of affecting other people—bringing smiles, joy and goodness out of them.

Emily finally finished her scoop of ice cream, and we went back to the marina to watch for Dave and Ryan. Once they finished their joy ride in the water, we went back to the house to get Sandy and do one final sweep. Then we would be back on the road to the comfort of our home.

The next day, back home, I brought Emily in for her scan. I hobbled her to the waiting room from the parking lot, and when her name was called, the technician brought a wheelchair for Emily to use. Emily, true to form, said, "I don't need the wheelchair. I can walk."

"Emily," I answered, "it's a good idea to use the chair."

"But I know how to walk, and I can walk," she resisted.

The technician interjected, "It is a far walk. I think you'll be more comfortable in the chair."

"Fine," she finally relented.

My shoulders relaxed with her sitting in the wheelchair. How amazingly easy it was to get to the MRI room when I wasn't balancing her every move. The MRI went fine, like it usually did. We drove home right after this time instead of meeting with the doctor, since this was a Saturday appointment.

That week I spoke with the neurologist again. She said the scans showed nothing remarkable. It was a bit difficult to explain her setbacks and what she was experiencing, but she would keep meeting with teams of doctors to try to figure it out. My head was swimming with the lack of answers, making me wonder if everything Emily was going through was just an illusion. I felt like an idiot when I had to explain why she suddenly couldn't walk without holding onto a counter, wall, or my hand for assistance. "We think she may have had a stroke. Honestly, we don't know why, you'll just need to hold her hand. And watch the drool." I kept clarifying to teachers or friends that we *were* taking her to doctors—they just didn't have an answer.

Emily was unloading the bottom rack of the dishwasher, as she liked to do, a few weeks after we were home from the beach. I didn't even know the dishwasher cycle had finished and she was unloading it; I just walked into the kitchen to watch her lose her balance and fall into the open dishwasher. She screamed, of course, sending Dave running into the kitchen. He pulled her out and asked if she was hurt.

"No," she said through tears.

I looked her up and down, and, other than a bruise forming on her leg, I didn't see anything else. I walked her to the couch to rest.

"Goddamnit!" I heard Dave yell in the kitchen. He was staring at our brand-new dishwasher, purchased one month earlier, smashed into pieces. "There's no way I can fix this!"

"Calm down. It was an accident," I told him.

"She's not allowed to unload the dishwasher anymore!" He was fuming.

He walked upstairs and slammed the door shut to our bedroom. I sat at the kitchen table and held back my tears. As angry as I was at

Dave for blowing up, I got it. I knew this was Dave having a moment. While I was quick to tears, he was quick to anger. So much was out of our control, and for someone who liked to be in control, like Dave, it was maddening.

Dave stayed locked away in our bedroom for the rest of the afternoon. I stayed away and let him stew. When he finally came downstairs, he asked Emily if she felt okay. She nodded her head. I told him we didn't have to get the dishwasher fixed right away—we could just hand wash the dishes for a while, thinking he was worried about the money it would cost to fix it.

"It's not about the dishwasher, Amy." He looked at me, defeated. "It's just this whole situation. It sucks."

We decided, after the dishwasher incident, Emily needed a wheelchair. She was a fall risk, even more than she was before. She couldn't be walking independently anymore. I dreaded lugging a chair in and out of a car, finding ramps, dealing with cracks and potholes in sidewalks, and finding the elevators in every building. But having a chair would mean that she could be safe, and it meant I didn't need to balance her every move. It allowed for some freedoms.

I called our social worker to learn the process, and the next thing I knew, we had a meeting set up at Emily's school to meet with her occupational therapist to take measurements and choose the proper type of chair. With this meeting around the corner, we needed to break the news to Emily.

"Guess what? We're going to get you your very own wheelchair to have at home!" I said in my most cheery voice.

She just looked at me, not buying my excited act.

"This means we can all go out together and you don't need to worry about getting tired. It will be so much easier!"

Her lip started to jut out.

"You only need to use it when we're out in stores and things like that. You can still walk at home." I was met with a stony silence. "You can pick whatever color wheelchair you want."

"I want pink."

When the chair arrived a month later, Emily smiled. She had picked a sparkly pink color and I told her that she was going to be so fancy, which made her beam. After I learned how to put it together and fold it and how the parts worked, she sat in it and asked, "Can you take my picture?"

"Sure!" I ran and grabbed my phone to take her picture. This was a long way from refusing to use a wheelchair. I guess it just needed to be pretty.

27

Answers

Emily and I met with a group of doctors from the neurology and autoimmune disorder clinics to discuss her recent setbacks. The result of this meeting was, of course, numerous orders for more tests.

I was happy that all these doctors were working to find out what exactly was going on, but I struggled with the underlying thought that it probably didn't matter. There was most likely nothing that could be done to fix anything. Should I continue to take her to these appointments if her health wouldn't change anyway? The stress and anxiety Emily had surrounding doctors' offices had only grown worse over time. Why put her through more?

After many discussions, Dave and I decided to do one non-invasive test at a time. The first one was a PET scan scheduled for Monday. We would see what it said before deciding to go on with the other testing.

The Saturday before that appointment, though, the neurologist called me.

"I cancelled the PET scan on Monday," she quickly told me.

"What? Why?"

"I presented Emily's case again at a conference last night, and there was a consensus that she's experiencing symptoms from radiation-induced vasculopathy. There was one doctor in particular who strongly believes, without a doubt, that is what Emily has. She's an incredible doctor with more than 20 years of experience. The others in the room agreed with her summary. There's no need to go forward with further testing."

"What is radiation-induced vasculopathy?" I asked, vaguely

remembering that Emily's epilepsy neurologist believed her to be suffering from that as well.

"It's damage to her arteries in her brain from the radiation treatment she had years ago. The symptoms tend to creep up about a decade out—which matches up with Emily's timing." She paused before adding, "There's no treatment for it. I'm really sorry."

"It's okay." I wasn't fully comprehending the diagnosis and especially the prognosis. I didn't want the doctor to feel sorry for me, though. She tried so hard to find answers regarding Emily's backward progression.

"I'm really so sorry," she repeated.

I stopped. I realized then that she was telling me that there was no cure and no getting better from this disease. How does one react to this news? I stayed silent, still comprehending, not fully believing.

"Do you want me to set up a meeting with the doctor who was very vocal about her diagnosis? She could probably answer any questions you have in more detail. She's a radiation oncologist for adults."

"Yes, please. I think that would be good."

I got off the phone and explained to Dave my conversation with the doctor. He was full of questions to which I didn't have the answers, but I wrote them down for my next meeting with the doctor. I didn't feel the satisfaction of knowing a diagnosis that I thought I would feel. I still felt uneasy and unsure. Now I was anxious to meet with the other doctor, who was more knowledgeable about this diagnosis.

The next day, as I sat in front of my work computer, changing gears like I so often had to do, I read an email explaining that another round of layoffs happened that morning. I then saw a 3 p.m. phone meeting request with an executive with whom I had never worked. Maybe this was it—perhaps the layoffs weren't done yet and I was next. There was no time to ponder, though, so I put the thought away, compartmentalizing it like I'd become so accustomed to doing, and started in on the mountain of emails that awaited me.

I paused at 2:30 when Emily came home from school. Mia was there to greet her, as well, and shortly after that I ran upstairs to have my 3 o'clock phone call with the executive.

"Hi, Amy. As you know, the company went through a reorganization this morning, and we'd like to move you to my department," the executive said to me.

"Okay," I said, used to being shuffled around to various departments and only a bit relieved I wasn't laid off.

"You'd report to the newly-created position of Director of Evaluations. I put Charles in that role, so you will be reporting to him."

My heart sank. For more than five years, I had been the only person responsible for evaluations at that company. Charles had only worked at the company for three years and in a completely different role. Beyond that, I was extremely more qualified than Charles for the position.

"Why did you put Charles in that role?" I finally asked.

"He's really enthusiastic. I've been working with him for a while now. I think he'll be great," he said.

"But I've been the one managing evaluations for five years. I have more than 20 years of experience managing surveys in my professional career," I told him.

"Well, I didn't know that. I mean, I don't even know you—this is our first conversation. Will this be a problem?"

"Yes, I won't work for Charles," I said in a shaky voice. I had never been so defiant at work, but I knew who Charles was and I didn't feel he operated with integrity. On multiple occasions he took my work and presented it at face-to-face meetings with executives without inviting me. He was also one to stay and schmooze after meetings while I ran home to be with Emily. *Dammit.*

"Fine, just report to me then. I really don't have time to manage people, though, so don't expect a lot of support. And our time is up—I've got to catch a flight. We can touch base in a few weeks." And he hung up.

I walked into Dave's office and burst into tears. I told him word for word what happened.

"Quit! Call him back and quit!"

I looked at Dave with desperation. I was so sad and angry, and yet it still wasn't easy for me to quit. "I get to work from home," I uttered to Dave through sobs, "and the money."

"We moved here so that you could stay home with the kids. Now more than ever it might be a good idea," he calmly reminded me and smiled.

I wiped away my tears. "I can't work for them anymore."

He laughed. "I've been telling you to quit for years. You put up with a lot more than I would have."

I went downstairs and drafted a resignation letter. Just as I wrapped it up, the social worker came to the door for her scheduled quarterly visit. I put on a smile and welcomed her inside. After she chatted with Emily and Mia, we went through the same routine. *What doctors did Emily visit and when during the last three months? May I see the wheelchair? What other services do you need? What are your goals for Emily?*

As soon as the social worker left, I emailed my resignation letter. I quit my job. With no new job lined up. I was equal parts terrified and liberated.

The next day, I woke up rehashing the events of the day before. Maybe I *will* just stay home. The holidays are coming up. The kids will have a lot of time off from school. I could finally be present and enjoy the time with them. Or maybe I'll look for a part-time job and try to get the best of both worlds. Before I made any other decisions, though, I wanted that meeting with the radiation oncologist.

Within a few weeks, Emily and I met the radiation oncologist who strongly believed Emily was suffering from radiation-induced vasculopathy. The doctor was kind and personable, and she spoke directly with Emily. She explained why she so passionately believed the diagnosis, having recognized the symptoms after working with radiation patients for 20 years. Plus, Emily's excessive radiation doses made her susceptible to the disease.

"Veins and arteries are supposed to be smooth," she explained, "but some of Emily's in her brain are rigid and crooked, like an old tree with branches in every direction, not allowing the blood to flow through properly. That results are those stroke-like episodes you've seen."

"So, the arteries are damaged from the radiation? Why is it just showing up now?" I asked, thinking how ironic it was that the treatment that once saved her life was now causing so much mayhem.

"Research has shown that about 10 years after treatment, some patients experience this. Emily's had a lot of treatment, which may have made her more likely to suffer from this."

"Is there anything we can do?" I asked, with little hope.

"No. The damage is irreversible and there's nothing we can do to stop it from further progressing."

There. She said it. Just like the other doctor. This can't be fixed. There was no going back to my old Emily. This wasn't quite news to me, but it was painful to hear nonetheless. Like a quick, sharp stab in my gut. I felt like I was shaking, but I looked down at my hands and they were still.

"So what should we expect? She had a stroke-like episode in April and another one in October. Will there be another one coming?" I wanted to know what lay ahead. I wanted to be prepared. I think I knew the outcome, but I would like the doctor to tell me exactly, in every detail available, what would happen next. I was so tired of surprises.

"My guess is yes, but I don't know when. It's likely that she's just in the early stages of this disease." She added, "So far the damage is to her little, tiny arteries. At some point it's likely to affect her larger veins and arteries. You would see something more serious at that point."

The outcome, she guessed, would be a life-threatening stroke. And we didn't know when that would occur or even if it would occur. Like her tumor, there was no predicting if or when it would grow. Another ticking time bomb.

The doctor couldn't, of course, predict our future, but she was giving me her best guess as to what might happen with Emily. Even though this news was devastating, I started to feel alarmingly at peace. I didn't tear up or cry. I smiled at Emily. She has endured so much and still managed to smile, laugh, and crack a joke. Even the doctor and her staff of interns and residents who visited with us that afternoon were blown away by how sweet and funny Emily was.

After reading her chart, the residents expected a shell of a person to be sitting in that wheelchair. Instead, they got someone who smiled, said hello, yelled at them that their hands were cold, and asked for chocolate for having to go to the doctor's office yet again. They met a girl who told them she was cooking dinner that night after she swept the floors when we got home. They were told that she and her best friend Mia were going to McDonald's that weekend for fries. She then told the doctors, complete with an eye roll, about her crazy brother who lies around and plays video games. No, she'd tell them, she doesn't like video games. But she plays the Wii, boasting about her bowling skills on Wii Sports, having once scored a perfect 300. They were then given a picture she drew of hearts, rainbows and flowers.

We ended the visit with smiles on our faces, and we were told to call if we needed anything. I had no meeting or email to rush home to. Instead, Emily and I chatted as we strolled to the car, me pushing her in her bright pink, sparkly wheelchair, talking about how nice those doctors were. We hit a traffic jam on the way home, at which point I turned the radio up and Emily and I sang at the top of our lungs.

That night, I made dinner, and the four of us sat at the table eating, talking and joking like we did most nights. Sandy sat under Dave waiting for scraps to be thrown her way. I wasn't a wreck. I wasn't stressed. I had no place I'd rather be. After Emily went to bed and Ryan plugged himself into the PlayStation, Dave and I took a walk. We talked through everything the doctor said. There were still many questions and what-ifs that we didn't have the answers to and probably never would.

In a strange way, we were suddenly free to live in the moment and not dwell on the unknown. After all, that's what Emily had been doing all along.

Epilogue

A few months of not working turned into a year of not working. I spent my days chauffeuring Ryan to his various activities, reminding him to do his homework, and playing catch with him in the backyard. I scheduled and coordinated all of Emily's appointments, took her to the doctors for routine check-ups and scans, and colored lots of pictures. Dave and I went out to lunch every week, had drinks with our neighbors, and walked miles and miles around the block, bringing our old dog, Sandy, along with us.

Emily's health is still full of ups and downs, and we are well aware it will always be like this. Her tumor, the damn thing that started this adventure, finally stabilized. It's still there, threatening to grow at any moment, but for now, it's quiet. Her Crohn's disease is well managed with a new medication, but there is concern she has developed an allergy to it because she now breaks out in hives for weeks at a time. Emily can go weeks without having a seizure, and then she will have four days in a row where she has two to three a day. Again, we don't know why or if there is a trigger. She had another stroke-like episode that they just termed a stroke. She recovered in the hospital for a few days, then came home and slipped right back into her regular routine.

I am at peace with Emily's mysterious ways. I don't feel the urge to figure out each medical malady that comes her way, and they are numerous. Instead, I concentrate on making her comfortable and don't waste more time than necessary figuring it out. She's a happy 20-year-old. She continues to draw pictures and play the Wii every day. Mia still comes over to hang out with her several days a week, and we still visit Nana and Grandpa for a good time.

Emily's world seems small, but she's content with the basic routine of our life. While her days may rarely change, Emily changes the lives of everyone she meets. She leaves anyone we come across with a smile, from the hairdresser she playfully "fired" because she didn't have any chocolate, to the McDonald's cashier Emily said looked pretty. Emily is not her body—she is the beautiful soul within it.

Ryan and Emily have a playful relationship and Ryan continues to be understanding of her and, therefore our, limitations. I finally broke it to Dave that I don't like vacationing. Taking Emily out of her routine is too much work, and I don't like waking up at 5 on vacations when I get to sleep until 6 at home. With that news, he and Ryan decided to make the father-son birthday trip an annual thing. They went to Colorado, Utah, and the Grand Canyon on their next trip and loved it.

I may eventually look for some part-time work to keep busy and add to our retirement fund, but I'm not in a hurry, and I'm not stressed out about it. Dark thoughts don't rattle in my brain anymore. I now think of them as freeing. Freeing for her and freeing for me. I lost my urge to be "normal" and to fit into the daily routines of the suburban families we are surrounded by. Instead of going to the movies to see the latest release, we watch *Lilo and Stitch* in our family room. We don't go to concerts and new restaurant openings. We let Emily go to bed at 7 and invite people to our house so we can have time with friends. I learned, from Emily, of course, to take each day as it comes and to smile and enjoy it.

⇒⊏   ⇒⊏   ⇒⊏

Emily passed away at the age of 21 in the summer of 2020. Although not unexpected, it was, of course, not an easy time. However, we took our cues and lessons learned from sweet Em and tried to stay positive as the days moved on.

Index

Numbers in **bold italics** indicate pages with illustrations